Push your Career Publish your Thesis

Science should be accessible to everybody. Share the knowledge, the ideas, and the passion about your research. Give your part of the infinite amount of scientific research possibilities a finite frame.

Publish your examination paper, diploma thesis, bachelor thesis, master thesis, dissertation, or habilitation treatises in form of a book.

A finite frame by infinite science.

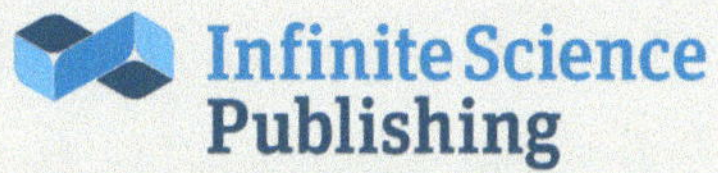

An Imprint of
Infinite Science GmbH
MFC 1 | Technikzentrum Lübeck
BioMedTec Wissenschaftscampus
Maria-Goeppert-Straße 1
23562 Lübeck
book@infinite-science.de
www.infinite-science.de

Editor

Thorsten M. Buzug
Institute of Medical Engineering
University of Lübeck
buzug@imt.uni-luebeck.de

Reihe: Medizinische Ingenieurwissenschaft und Biomedizintechnik

Diese Reihe umfasst Werke der Medizinischen Ingenieurwissenschaft und Biomedizintechnik, deren Themen strategisch unter den Zukunftstechnologien mit hohem Innovationspotenzial anzusiedeln sind. Als wesentliche Trends dieser Forschungsgebiete, sind die Schlüsselbereiche Computerisierung, Miniaturisierung und Molekularisierung zu nennen. Bei der Computerisierung sind dabei die inhaltlichen Schwerpunkte beispielsweise in der Bildgebung und Bildverarbeitung gegeben. Die Miniaturisierung spielt unter anderem bei intelligenten Implantaten, der minimalinvasiven Chirurgie aber auch bei der Entwicklung von neuen nanostrukturierten Materialien eine wichtige Rolle, und die Molekularisierung ist in der regenerativen Medizin aber auch im Rahmen der sogenannten molekularen Bildgebung ein entscheidender Aspekt. Forschungs- und Entwicklungspotenzial werden auch der Biophotonik und der minimal-invasiven Chirurgie unter Berücksichtigung der Robotik und Navigation zugeschrieben. Querschnittstechnologien wie die Mikrosystemtechnik, optische Technologien, Softwaresysteme und Wissenstechnologien sind dabei von hohem Interesse.

Christina Kluck

Pharyngeal Airflow Simulation in Obstructive Sleep Apnea Patients

Medical Engineering Science and Biomedical Engineering — Volume 7

Editor: Thorsten M. Buzug

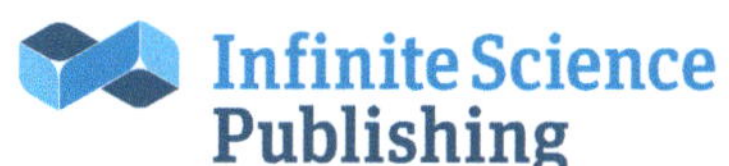

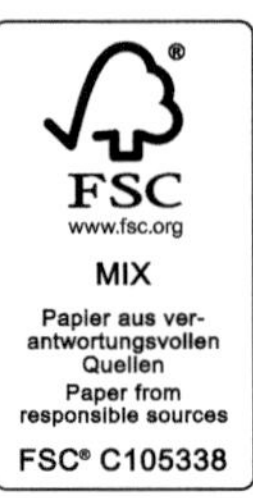

Abstract

The airflow to the lungs is disturbed by a partial or complete collapse of the upper airways
of patients suffering from Obstructive Sleep Apnea. Numerical simulations on patient specific
models may be used to extract pathophysiological parameters like flow velocity and pressure
distribution in the human pharynx and can evaluate the severity of the disease and the success
of a therapy. Within this work Computational Fluid Dynamics (CFD) are used to simulate the
airflow in the natural pharyngeal geometry of a patient as well as in the deformed pharyngeal
geometry of the same patient treated with a dental appliance. The simulations are performed
with two different types of boundary conditions to investigate the influence of the choice of
boundary conditions. It is found that a realistic choice of a pressure drop boundary condition
shows a significant change in the pressure distribution for the different geometries. In using an
inflow velocity as boundary condition a change in the dimensionless Reynolds number based on
the flow velocity can be observed.
A comparison of two different turbulence models showed no significant differences in the flow
predictions.

Kurzfassung

Schlafapnoepatienten leiden darunter, dass der Luftstrom zur Lunge gestört ist aufgrund von
kollabierenden Atemwegen im Rachenraum. Mittels numerischer Simulationen können an pa-
tientenspezifischen Modellen pathopysiologische Parameter wie die Strömungsgeschwindigkeit
und die Druckverteilung gewonnen und benutzt werden, um Schweregrad der Erkrankung und
Erfolg einer Therapie zu evaluieren. In dieser Arbeit werden numerische Strömungsberechnungen
sowohl an der originalen Rachengeometrie eines Schlafapnoepatienten als auch an einer durch
eine Dentalschiene veränderten Rachengeometrie desselben Patienten vorgenommen. Für diese
Simulationen werden zwei unterschiedliche Arten von Randbedingungen gewählt, um die Aus-
wirkungen der Auswahl von Randbedingungen zu untersuchen. Dabei zeigt sich, dass eine
physikalisch realistische Wahl von Druckabfallsrandbedingungen eine signifikante Änderung in
der Druckverteilung aufweist für die unterschiedlichen Rachengeometrien. Benutzt man eine
Einströmgeschwindigkeit als Randbedingung, so kann eine Änderung in der auf der Strömungsgeschwindigkeit basierenden dimensionslosen Reynoldszahl beobachtet werden.
Der Vergleich von zwei unterschiedlichen Turbulenzmodellen wies keine signifikanten Änderungen
in den Strömungsvorhersagen auf.

Contents

1 Introduction   1

2 Basics   5
  2.1 Partial Differential Equations   5
  2.2 Computational Fluid Dynamics   9
      2.2.1 Mathematical Model   10
      2.2.2 Finite Element Method   22
      2.2.3 Numerical Solution   26
      2.2.4 Accuracy of CFD   33

3 Material and Methods   35
  3.1 Preprocessing   35
  3.2 Simulation   41
  3.3 Experimental Validation   47

4 Results   49
  4.1 Comparison to Measurement   49
  4.2 Pharyngeal Flow Simulation   56
      4.2.1 Grid Dependency   56
      4.2.2 Comparison of patient data   67

5 Discussion   75
  5.1 Comparison to Measurement   75
  5.2 Comparison of Patient Data   75
  5.3 Reliability of the Models   76

6 Conclusion and Outlook   79

7 Appendix   81

1 Introduction

2% of women and 4% of men in the middle-aged American population suffer from the Obstructive Sleep Apnea Hypopnea Syndrome (OSAHS) [80]. The patient's upper airways are partially (hypopnea) or completely (apnea) closed leading to a breathing disorder during sleep. The upper

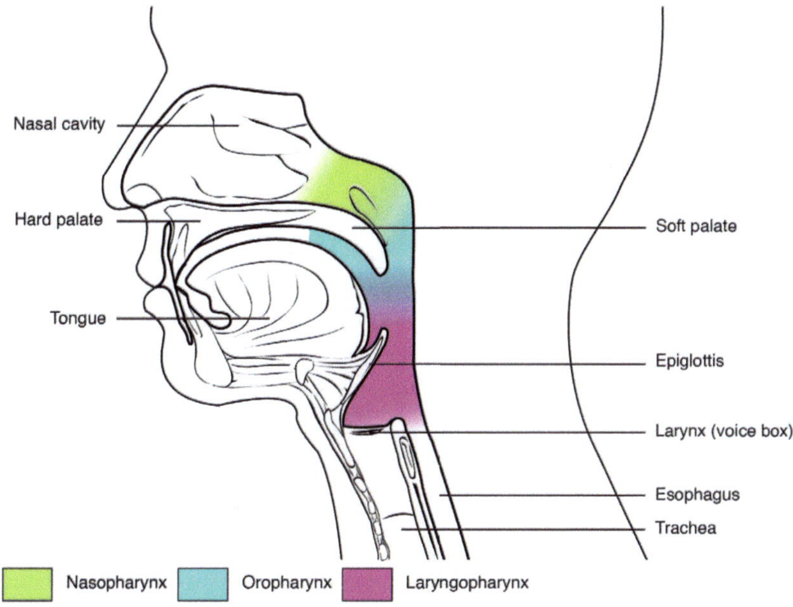

Figure 1.1: Obstruction may take place in the human's upper airway system, more precisely in the pharynx, which is formed by the nasopharynx, oropharynx and laryngopharynx. The image is taken from [56].

airway consists of four parts: the nasal cavity, the pharynx, the larynx and the trachea, as can be seen in figure 1.1. Sleep related obstructions can occur at the level of the pharynx, which is a pipe-like structure formed by muscles. The pharynx is not bound by bony structures so that it is collapsible at the area between the hard palate and the larynx. During the sleep the tone of the pharyngeal muscles is reduced, which may result in the collapse of the pharynx. There are several factors narrowing the pharyngeal lumen predisposing the patient to suffer from OS-AHS. Among these are structural and anatomical factors constricting the pharyngeal soft tissue like maxilla or mandibular malformations and soft tissue enlargements caused by hypertrophied tonsils, adenoids and tongue or the fat deposition by a patient suffering from obesity.
OSAHS patients show a characteristic snoring pattern of alternating load snoring and silence. In the apneic series a brake off of respiration occurs and the upper airway muscles have to be activated to restore the airflow to the lungs. These cessations can cause an insufficient alveolar ventilation resulting in a reduction of oxygen saturation and arousals from the patient's sleep

[3], [4], [63], [24].

The main daytime symptom is excessive sleepiness. OSAHS is often accompanied with a reduction in life quality, even a correlation with depression is reported [67]. In [46] and [57] a linear correspondence between the severity of OSAHS and hypertension is found and it is asserted that OSAHS can serve as a significant independent predictor of cardiopulmonary death. Yaggi et al. [79] declared that OSAHS increases the risk of stroke and death.

Hence, OSAHS represents a disease that not only affects the patient's life quality in a negative way but also impairs his state of health.

The standard treatment for OSAHS patients is the Continuous Positive Airway Pressure (CPAP). The patient's pharynx should be prevented from collapsing by a constant positive pressure established by a mask the patient is wearing during sleep. But a life-long application of the pressure mask every night is not suitable for all patients. Boudewyns et al. [8] reported that poor treatment compliance and/or refusal is an issue for 20–30 % of the patients. A non-invasive alternative treatment method is the wearing of a dental mandibular repositioning device that is intended to widen the pharyngeal lumen by soft tissue deformations resulting from the repositioning of the jaw. Other non-invasive treatments are rare, Puhan et al. [58] describe that didgeridoo playing may ease OSAHS symptoms. They assume the reason in the training of the airway muscles.

If no non-invasive treatment is suitable, OSAHS patients are either treated with a reduction of soft tissue in the upper airway called Uvulopalatopharyngoplasty (UPPP) and/or the surgical repositioning of the jaw, which is in general an advancement of the mandibular called Maxillomandibular Advancement Osteotomy (MMO). The surgical treatment is often performed in a step-wise manner, so that the UPPP is the phase 1 intervention and if it is not sufficient the phase 2 intervention can be the MMO surgery.

Bettega et al. [7] studied the success of both surgical treatments, UPPP and MMO. They concluded that UPPP has a success rate of only 22.7 %. And also the second phase the MMO surgery was found to leave 25 % of the examined patients with an unsuccessful outcome.

This work is part of a project targeting at the simulation of the deformation of an individual patient's pharyngeal geometry evoked by surgical mandibular repositioning or dental appliances. Numerical simulations of the airflow in digitized models of the original and the simulated deformed geometry shall be performed to examine the differences in the airflow dynamics caused by the surgical treatment or the appliance respectively. It is assumed that the success of the therapy can be evaluated by comparison of the different flow situations. That would imply a great benefit, because an optimal individual therapy planning could be provided that prevents unnecessary surgical interventions risking the patient's health. Concerning a surgical method which does not provide the desired outcome in 25 % of all treatments an evaluation of the result a-priori to the intervention is desirable. Furthermore in-silico simulations of soft tissue deformations and resulting fluid dynamics could make it possible to identify the optimal mandibular position with respect to the outcome of the treatment. In the case of treatment with a mandibular advancement appliance the influence of the device's shape on the severity of the disease could be evaluated without producing the device. The patient individual design of an optimal shape could become possible.

Within this project this work deals with the aspect of the airflow simulation. Two cone beam computed tomography datasets of one patient suffering from OSAHS are used for the flow analysis. One of the datasets is obtained with the patient wearing a mandibular advancement appliance (MAA) causing a deformation of the pharyngeal geometry and the other dataset is obtained without any treatment showing the natural pharyngeal geometry. Hence, the comparison of natural and deformed geometry is possible.

The principles that can be used for the numerical simulation of airflow are summarized under the denomination *Computational Fluid Dynamics*. A fluid is a material that holds no resistance to applied shear forces, mainly that are liquids and gases so as air [27]. The motion of fluids can be described using certain equations called Navier Stokes Equations (NSE) that are derived from fundamental conservation principles and fluid's parameters like its density and viscosity. Flow dynamics of fluids like air can be predicted by the numerical solution of the Navier Stokes Equations for the velocity and the pressure in a prescribed computational domain.

Computational Fluid Dynamics have already been used to examine pathophysiological parameters corresponding to constrictions in the human upper airway. It was found by flow simulations in idealized models of the upper airways that a significant pressure drop occurs in the narrowest regions and that the flow within human pharynx is in the laminar-to-turbulent transitional flow regime [61], [69], [48]. Li et al. [48] confirmed their simulation results with an experimental measurement in the idealized human pharyngeal geometry. Shome et al. [69] concluded that a slight change in the pharynx geometry caused by a mandibular surgery might effect the flow profile significantly because of the transitional state of the flow in the constricted pharynx. In using patient specific models gained by computer tomographic or magnet resonance tomographic data it was confirmed by several authors with fluid simulations, that a treatment of OSAHS either with a surgery or a dental appliance leads to reduction in the pressure drop along the investigated pharynx [77], [26], [53], [39], [73], [74].

Often models are used in simulating turbulent flow which describe turbulent effects. In many cases the $k - \epsilon$ model or a low Reynolds number version of it is used, for example in [26], [53], [61], [48]. Within this work two different turbulence models, the standard $k - \epsilon$ turbulence model and the $k - \omega$ turbulence model, are used for the simulations. They divide in the aspect that the $k - \epsilon$ model uses a turbulence parameter called dissipation, which describes the rate at which kinetic energy is transformed into thermal energy. The $k - \omega$ turbulence model is despite the $k - \epsilon$ model one of the most used turbulence models in the area of Computational Fluid Dynamics [76]. Instead of the dissipation the specific dissipation rate is modeled in the $k - \omega$ model. The specific dissipation rate is the ratio of dissipation to the turbulence intensity. The two different models are known to perform differently in some flow phenomena modelings [76]. Within this work the flow is modeled using both mentioned turbulence models to investigate, if differences arise in the predicted flows.

For the simulation of fluid flow dynamics it is necessary to prescribe some conditions on the computational boundaries. In most of the cases the flow inlet is prescribed with an inflow velocity or a volume inflow rate [26], [61], [69], [48], [73]. In [74] a different kind of boundary condition is used: a prescribed pressure drop between inflow inlet and outlet. Is is justified with the physical reflection of the lung establishing a pressure drop in the human respiratory system during inspiration. Within this work both described types of boundary conditions are used and the simulations are investigated concerning differences in the simulates velocities and pressures. Within this work simulations of fluid flow are performed in the original as well as in the deformed geometry, the flow profile and the pressure distribution of the different geometries is compared to examine the relevance of this quantities for the prediction of OSAHS severity. Special attention is paid to the different aspects of a fluid flow simulation task, like the dependency of the achieved solution on the used computational grid and the choice of prescribed boundary conditions on the flow. The computations are performed using a multiphysics simulation tool based on finite element modeling COMSOL©, provided by COMSOL Inc. [36]

In the first chapter of this work the basics of partial differential equations are given, because the equations needed for simulating fluid flow are of that type. In the same chapter an introduction to Computational Fluid Dynamics is given. Chapter 3 describes how the medical datasets are transferred into digital models, on which fluid flow simulations are performed. Experimental data of a similar medical task, a model of a constricted artery, is compared to simulation results for validating reasons. In chapter 4 the results are presented, which are discussed in chapter 5. In chapter 6 a conclusion and outlook on future work is given.

2 Basics

2.1 Partial Differential Equations

Partial Differential Equations (PDEs) are often used in physics for modeling purposes. PDEs describe the change of a physical quantity in relation to several independent variables like the propagation of a spherical wave depending on its velocity (time derivative) and its shape (spatial derivative).
A PDE is an equation which involves an unknown function $u : \Omega \subseteq \mathbb{R}^d \to \mathbb{R}$ and some of its partial derivatives. Here, a scalar valued function is regarded for simplicity reasons, but derived concepts are also applicable to vector valued functions.
Within this chapter the following notation conventions are used:

- A vector $\alpha = (\alpha_1, ..., \alpha_d)$ with $\alpha_i \in \mathbb{N}$ is called a *multiindex* of *order*

$$|\alpha| = \alpha_1 + \cdots + \alpha_d. \tag{2.1}$$

- Regarding a multiindex α

$$D^\alpha u(\boldsymbol{x}) := \frac{\partial^{|\alpha|} u(\boldsymbol{x})}{\partial x_1^{\alpha_1} \cdots \partial x_n^{\alpha_n}} = \partial_{x_1}^{\alpha_1} \cdots \partial_{x_n}^{\alpha_n} u \tag{2.2}$$

  is defined.

- The set of all partial derivatives of order $k \in \mathbb{N}$ is then given by

$$D^k u(\boldsymbol{x}) := \{ D^\alpha u(\boldsymbol{x}) \mid |\alpha| = k \}. \tag{2.3}$$

The explanations follow mainly [25].

Definition 2.1 *Given an open subset $\Omega \subseteq \mathbb{R}^d$, a function $u : \Omega \to \mathbb{R}$ and the independent variable $\boldsymbol{x} = (x_1, ..., x_d) \in \Omega$. An equation of the form*

$$\mathcal{L}u = F(D^k u(\boldsymbol{x}), D^{k-1} u(\boldsymbol{x}), ..., Du(\boldsymbol{x}), u(\boldsymbol{x}), \boldsymbol{x}) = 0 \tag{2.4}$$

with

$$F =: \mathbb{R}^{d^k} \times \mathbb{R}^{d^{k-1}} \times \cdots \times \mathbb{R}^d \times \mathbb{R} \times \Omega \to \mathbb{R}$$

is called a kth-order ordinary differential equation if only derivatives of one component x_i appear and k^{th}-order partial differential equation otherwise.

There is no overall treatment for all partial differential equations, but PDEs are subdivided in characteristic groups which show similar behavior.

Definition 2.2 *For given functions $a_\alpha(|\alpha| \leq k), f$ PDE (2.4) is called*

(i) linear, *if it has the form*

$$\sum_{|\alpha| \leq k} a_\alpha(\boldsymbol{x}) D^\alpha u = f(\boldsymbol{x}),$$

homogeneous *in the case $f \equiv 0$,*

(ii) semilinear, *if it has the form*

$$\sum_{|\alpha|=k} a_\alpha(\boldsymbol{x}) D^\alpha u + a_0(D^{k-1}u, ..., Du, u, \boldsymbol{x}) = 0,$$

(iii) quasilinear, *if it has the form*

$$\sum_{|\alpha|=k} a_\alpha(D^{k-1}u, ..., Du, u, \boldsymbol{x}) + a_0(D^{k-1}u, ..., Du, u, \boldsymbol{x}) = 0,$$

(iv) fully nonlinear *if it depends nonlinearly on the kth order derivatives.*

A function u is called solution, if it satisfies equation (2.4) in every point $x \in \Omega$. Auxiliary boundary conditions are demanded on u on some part Γ on the boundary $\partial\Omega$ of Ω to define one unique solution. There are two types of boundary conditions for $\partial\Omega = \Gamma_D \cup \Gamma_N$ with $\Gamma_D \cap \Gamma_N = \emptyset$ and given functions $u_l : U \to \mathbb{R}, l \in \{D, N\}$

$$u = u_D \text{ on } \Gamma_D \tag{2.5a}$$
$$\partial_n u = u_N \text{ on } \Gamma_N \tag{2.5b}$$

with $n \in \mathbb{R}^d$, $||n||_2 = 1$ the normalized unit vector on the boundary $\partial\Omega$ pointing to $\Omega^c = \mathbb{R}^d \backslash \Omega$. (2.5a) is called *Dirichlet's boundary conditions* and (2.5b) *Neumann's boundary conditions*, in the special case of $u_N = 0$ they are named *homogeneous Neumann's boundary conditions*. In PDE problems resulting of physical applications often time t represents one of the independent variables and conditions on the unknown function u are demanded on an initial time point t_0. In that case the conditions are named initial value conditions. If they appear together with boundary conditions the problem is called an initial boundary value problem.

After Hadamard [32] a problem is well-posed, if it fulfills three conditions:

- There exists a solution to the problem,

- this solution is unique and

- the solution depends continuously on the data.

The problem is called ill-posed, if one or more of these conditions are not provided. The choice of the boundary conditions has influence on a problem involving PDEs of being well- or ill-posed [62]. A classification of PDEs in the categories *hyperbolic*, *parabolic* and *elliptic* can aid to distinguish boundary conditions leading to a well-posed problem. This distinction is entire for the linear second-order partial differential equation with the general form regarding a two dimensional space $\Omega \subseteq \mathbb{R}^2$

$$c_6 \, u_{x_1 x_1} + c_5 \, u_{x_1 x_2} + c_4 \, u_{x_2 x_2} + c_3 \, u_{x_1} + c_2 \, u_{x_2} + c_1 \, u + c_0, \tag{2.6}$$

with functions $c_i : \Omega \to \mathbb{R}, i \in \{0, ..., 6\}$.

Definition 2.3 *A partial differential equation of the form (2.6) is called*

(i) elliptic *in* (x_1, x_2), *if*

$$4\,c_6(x_1, x_2)\,c_4(x_1, x_2) - c_5^2(x_1, x_2) > 0$$

(ii) hyperbolic *in* (x_1, x_2), *if*

$$4\,c_6(x_1, x_2)\,c_4(x_1, x_2) - c_5^2(x_1, x_2) < 0$$

(iii) parabolic *in* (x_1, x_2), *if*

$$4\,c_6(x_1, x_2)\,c_4(x_1, x_2) - c_5^2(x_1, x_2) = 0 \quad and \quad rank \begin{bmatrix} c_6 & \frac{c_5}{2} & c_3 \\ \frac{c_5}{2} & c_4 & c_2 \end{bmatrix} = 2$$

(iv) elliptic (hyperbolic, parabolic) *in* Ω, *if it is* elliptic (hyperbolic, parabolic) *in every* $(x_1, x_2) \in \Omega$.

Elliptic PDEs The *Poisson's equation*

$$\partial_x^2 u(x, t) = f(x, t) \quad \forall (x, t) \in \Omega \subset \mathbb{R}^2 \tag{2.7}$$

is a characteristic example for a PDE of the elliptic type with two independent variables. For the special case of $f(x, t) \equiv 0$ it is called the *Laplace equation*. Elliptic PDEs need the definition of Dirichlet's or Neumann's boundary conditions on a closed region, hence on every part of the boundary. The different behavior of the three classes of PDEs can additionally be observed in the distribution of information. Regarding an elliptic PDE problem one point (x', t') distributes information in the whole area Ω and reversely every point of the solution is affected by a change somewhere on the whole boundary.

Parabolic PDEs The *heat equation*

$$\partial_t u(x, t) - \partial_x^2 u(x, t) = 0 \quad \forall (x, t) \in \Omega \subset \mathbb{R}^2. \tag{2.8}$$

is an example of a parabolic PDE. Dirichlet's or Neumann's boundary conditions have to be prescribed on an open region, hence the definition of boundary conditions is not allowed on the whole boundary $\partial \Omega$. Information is distributed from a point (x', t') the propagation direction $t \geq t'$. The solution in that point is affected by changes on the boundary, where $t \leq t'$ is valid.

Hyperbolic PDEs The *wave equation*

$$\partial_t^2 u(x, t) - \partial_x^2 u(x, t) = 0 \quad \forall (x, t) \in \Omega \subset \mathbb{R}^2 \tag{2.9}$$

is a prototype PDE of hyperbolic characteristic. It needs the definition of both the value and the slope of the function as condition on an open region, hence the definition of boundary conditions is not allowed on the whole boundary $\partial \Omega$. One point spreads information only along a certain cone. Points outside this cone are not affected by a change on that point.

Figure 2.1 shows schematically the distribution of information of the three classes, to visualize the area of influence that a certain point $(x', t') \in \Omega$ has on the resulting solution u. The point-wise classification *elliptic*, *hyperbolic* and *parabolic* can be expanded on second-order linear PDEs

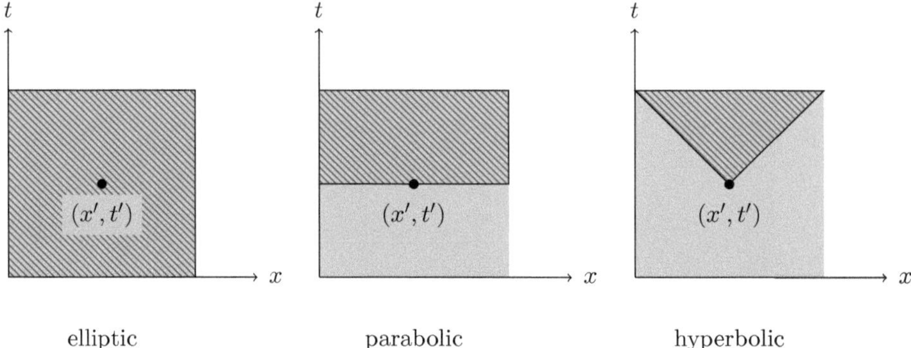

elliptic   parabolic   hyperbolic

Figure 2.1: The area of influence of one point (x', t') on the solution u of a partial differential equation is dependent on the class.

of more than two independent variables (see for example [31]) and also on higher order and quasi as well as semilinear PDEs by so called characteristic surfaces of the differential operator, see [62] for further information. In the following section the classification of the partial differential equations of interest within this context is presented.

Partial differential equations are sometimes converted to the so called *weak from* or *variational from*. The idea is to derive a formulation of the partial differential equations demanding less regularity of the solution than the original or *strong form*, which is important for discretization reasons. The weak form still preserves that a solution of the strong form is also a solution to the weak form. More information can be found in [47]. The derivation of the weak form of a PDE is exemplary shown using the PDE

$$\Delta \cdot \Gamma(u) = F(u) \quad u \in \Omega \tag{2.10}$$

with arbitrary boundary conditions. If a solution u fulfills this equation the same solution will still hold if we multiply (2.10) by any function $\tilde{u}$ called *test function* from a so called test space V providing that the test function $\tilde{u}$ is not zero and fulfills the demanded boundary conditions:

$$\Delta \cdot \Gamma(u) \cdot \tilde{u} = F(u) \cdot \tilde{u}.$$

Equality still holds if the resulting equation is then integrated over the computational domain Ω and by using Gauss' divergence theorem the differentiation can be shifted to the test function $\tilde{u}$ resulting in the weak form of the example PDE (2.10)

$$0 = \int_{\Omega} \nabla \tilde{u} \cdot \Gamma(u) - \tilde{u} F(u) \, \mathrm{d}\Omega, \tag{2.11}$$

see [60] for further details. Now the demands on the regularity of the solution u are reduced because of the shift of the differentiation which is useful for the discretization process concerning for example piecewise polynomial functions. The solution u must hold equation (2.11) for any arbitrary test function $\tilde{u} \in V$. In the process of discretization a solution $u \in V$ is searched for, that means the test function space also spans the solution space. Hence, by choosing a test function space V the quality of the numerical approximation is influenced.

The Finite Element Method (FEM) is an often used numerical scheme for the discretization of

PDEs. The weak form of an PDE is the base for the spatial discretization technique of FEM which section 2.2.2 deals with.

2.2 Computational Fluid Dynamics

Computation Fluid Dynamics (CFD) describe numerical simulation in the area of fluid mechanics. It arose within the area of engineering as a link between fluid mechanics theory and experimental results. CFD is targeted at giving numerical approximated (*computational*) predictions of fluid flow phenomena (*fluid dynamics*). A *fluid* is characterized by molecular structures holding no resistance to applied shear forces [27], so it deforms continually under applied shear stresses. Those substances are mainly liquids and gases. In most cases they can be regarded as a continuum. Fluids can be subdivided into *incompressible* fluids, which are mass preserving and volume preserving and *compressible* fluids, which are mass preserving but **not** volume preserving. Although most gases like air are compressible fluids, they are often considered as incompressible if the density change is small. The fluid's Mach number

$$\mathrm{Ma} = \frac{u}{a}, \tag{2.12}$$

where u describes the fluid's flow velocity and a the sound-propagation velocity within the fluid, is regarded to quantify the relevance of compressibility effects. In [27] fluid flow is said to act incompressible for $\mathrm{Ma} < 0.3$ and compressible in the contrary case. Although compressibility is a fluid's property the fluid flow is often called either compressible or incompressible depending on its behavior. Flows with $\mathrm{Ma} < 1$ where the fluid flows slower than its sound-propagation velocity are called *subsonic*. For $\mathrm{Ma} > 1$ the flow can contain shock waves, the flow is called *supersonic*. If the flow is very fast in relation to its sound-propagation velocity the compression may cause that high temperature that it changes the chemical nature of the fluid. This may be the case for $\mathrm{Ma} > 5$ where the flow is named *hypersonic*.

In general three steps have to be taken to simulate fluid dynamics:

Mathematical Model
> The starting point for the simulation of fluid dynamics is a mathematical model describing the physics and behavior of a fluid. In the present case a set of partial differential equations (PDEs) called the Navier Stokes Equations combined with boundary conditions are used to describe the flow mathematically.

Discretization
> In most cases the differential equations of the mathematical model are too complex to be solved analytically. They are approximated by a system of algebraic equations at a set of discrete points in space and time.

Numerical Solution
> The last step is the solution of the system of algebraic equations which is performed either by direct or iterative solver algorithms.

The composition of this chapter is orientated at the subdivision of the tasks in fluid dynamics computing. Section 2.2.1 draws the deduction of the Navier Stokes Equations based on conservative laws and introduces some models targeted on turbulent flows. There are three discretization techniques which are in wide spread usage to discretize PDE problems: Finite Volume Method, Finite Difference Method and Finite Element Method. Within this work the last one is used. It is introduced in section 2.2.2. The last section 2.2.3 of this chapter presents the steps from the discretized algebraic system to a numerical solution of the fluid dynamics problem.

2.2.1 Mathematical Model

This section deals with the Navier Stokes Equations named after Claude Louis Marie Henri Navier and George Gabriel Stokes, who formulated independently this law of fluid motion for so called *Newtonian* fluids.

Newtonian Fluid *A fluid is said to be Newtonian, if the resulting shear stress is linearly dependent on the shear rate. If the functional relation is non-linear the fluid is called Non-Newtonian.* [55]

Most gases are Newtonian fluids, examples for Non-Newtonian fluids are blood and ketchup. Within this context simulations of airflow are of interest. For air as a Newtonian fluid the Navier Stokes Equations are valid.

Navier Stokes Equations

This sections aims at deriving the Navier Stokes Equations of fluid motion by fundamental conservation principles. The explanations follow the illustrations in [27].
The conservation of a physical property can either be described regarding a given quantity of matter called *control mass* (CM) or in a certain spatial region, the *control volume* (CV). In the control mass description the property is dependent on the size of matter and is called an *extensive* property. In the case of control volume approach the properties are called *intensive*. Whereas the control mass approach is adequate to describe dynamics of solid bodies, it is difficult to follow a certain entity of matter in a fluid flow. Applying the CV approach a spatial region of interest is regarded instead. The different approaches are comparable. Let ϕ stand for any conserved intensive property, then the corresponding extensive property Φ can be determined by

$$\Phi = \int_{\Omega_{\mathrm{CM}}} \rho\phi \, \mathrm{d}\Omega, \tag{2.13}$$

where Ω_{CM} is the volume occupied by the corresponding control mass and ρ is the density.
In general the rate of change of a physical property is of interest. For any property ϕ the rate of change can be expressed using (2.13) by

$$\frac{\mathrm{d}}{\mathrm{d}t} \int_{\Omega_{\mathrm{CM}}} \rho\phi \, \mathrm{d}\Omega = \frac{\partial}{\partial t} \int_{\Omega_{\mathrm{CV}}} \rho\phi \, \mathrm{d}\Omega + \int_{\partial\Omega_{\mathrm{CV}}} \rho\phi\, \boldsymbol{u} \cdot \boldsymbol{n} \, \mathrm{d}s. \tag{2.14}$$

The control volume is denoted by Ω_{CV} and its surface by $\partial\Omega_{\mathrm{CV}}$. The unit vector $\boldsymbol{n}$ is orthogonal to the surface and directing outwards, $\boldsymbol{u}$ is the fluid velocity vector. The balance principle (2.14) states that the rate of change of the amount of a physical property within a control mass is the same as its rate of change in the control volume plus the net flux through the volume's boundary. The conservation principles addressed within this context are the conservation of mass

$$\frac{\mathrm{d}m}{\mathrm{d}t} = 0, \tag{2.15}$$

where m is the mass, and the conservation of momentum, also known as Newton's second law of motion

$$\frac{\mathrm{d}m\boldsymbol{u}}{\mathrm{d}t} = \sum \boldsymbol{f}, \tag{2.16}$$

where $\boldsymbol{f}$ denotes forces acting on the control mass. Both equations are given in the control mass description. In the following the control volume approach is considered, therefore the index notation is omitted, Ω denotes the control volume and $\partial\Omega$ its surface. With relation (2.14) the control volume formulation of the conservation principles can be derived. In the case of mass conservation the variable ϕ has just to be replaced by $\phi = 1$ resulting in

$$\frac{\partial}{\partial t}\int_{\Omega} \rho\,\mathrm{d}\Omega + \int_{\partial\Omega} \rho\boldsymbol{u}\cdot\boldsymbol{n}\,\mathrm{d}s = 0. \tag{2.17}$$

In usage of the Gauss' divergence theorem[1] and an infinitesimal small control volume Ω

$$\frac{\partial\rho}{\partial t} + \nabla\cdot(\rho\boldsymbol{u}) = 0 \tag{2.18}$$

is derived, where $\nabla = \left(\frac{\partial}{\partial x}, \frac{\partial}{\partial y}, \frac{\partial}{\partial z}\right)^T$ is the vector of spatial derivative operators.

By applying (2.14) to the conservation principle of momentum, ϕ has to be replaced by $\phi = \boldsymbol{u}$ to get

$$\frac{\partial}{\partial t}\int_{\Omega} \rho\boldsymbol{u}\,\mathrm{d}\Omega + \int_{\partial\Omega} \rho\boldsymbol{u}\boldsymbol{u}\cdot\boldsymbol{n}\,\mathrm{d}s = \sum\boldsymbol{f}. \tag{2.19}$$

There are two different types of forces acting on the control volume in the area of fluid dynamics:

- body forces $\boldsymbol{f}_b$ (like gravity and electromagnetic forces, etc.) and

- surface forces $\boldsymbol{f}_s$ (like surface tension and pressure, etc.).

If $\boldsymbol{b}$ represents body forces per unit mass the contribution of body forces can be determined by $\boldsymbol{f}_b = \int_{\Omega} \rho\boldsymbol{b}\,\mathrm{d}\Omega$.

The surface forces can be described using the stress tensor for Newtonian fluids

$$\mathbf{T} = -\left(p + \frac{2}{3}\mu\nabla\cdot\boldsymbol{u}\right)\mathbf{I} + 2\mu\mathbf{D}, \tag{2.20}$$

where μ is the dynamic viscosity, $\mathbf{I}$ is the unit tensor, p the static pressure and $\mathbf{D}$ is the rate of strain or deformation tensor

$$\mathbf{D} = \frac{1}{2}\left[\nabla\boldsymbol{u} + (\nabla\boldsymbol{u})^T\right]. \tag{2.21}$$

The contribution of surface forces can be derived by $\boldsymbol{f}_s = \int_{\partial\Omega} \mathbf{T}\cdot\boldsymbol{n}\,\mathrm{d}s$. Inserting $\boldsymbol{f}_b$ and $\boldsymbol{f}_s$ in (2.19) leads to

$$\frac{\partial}{\partial t}\int_{\Omega} \rho\boldsymbol{u}\,\mathrm{d}\Omega + \int_{\partial\Omega} \rho\boldsymbol{u}\boldsymbol{u}\cdot\boldsymbol{n}\,\mathrm{d}s = \int_{\partial\Omega} \mathbf{T}\cdot\mathrm{d}s + \int_{\Omega} \rho\boldsymbol{b}\,\mathrm{d}\Omega. \tag{2.22}$$

Again Gauss' theorem and infinitesimal small Ω are used, resulting in

$$\frac{\partial(\rho\boldsymbol{u})}{\partial t} + \rho\boldsymbol{u}\cdot\nabla\boldsymbol{u} = \nabla\cdot\mathbf{T} + \rho\boldsymbol{b}. \tag{2.23}$$

Together with the mass conservation (2.18) the Navier Stokes Equations for compressible, isothermal flow of Newtonian fluids are given by

$$\frac{\partial(\rho\boldsymbol{u})}{\partial t} + \rho\boldsymbol{u}\cdot\nabla\boldsymbol{u} = -\nabla p + \nabla\cdot\left[\mu\left(\nabla\boldsymbol{u} + (\nabla\boldsymbol{u})^T\right) - \frac{2}{3}\mu\left(\nabla\cdot\boldsymbol{u}\right)\mathbf{I}\right] + \rho\boldsymbol{b}$$

$$\frac{\partial\rho}{\partial t} + \nabla\cdot(\rho\boldsymbol{u}) = 0, \tag{2.24}$$

---

[1] Gauss' divergence theorem for a compact volume Ω with piecewise smooth boundary $\partial\Omega$ and continuously differentiable vector field $\mathbf{F}$: $\int_{\partial\Omega} \mathbf{F}\cdot\boldsymbol{n} = \int_{\Omega} \nabla\cdot\mathbf{F}$

which is a set of non-linear second order partial differential equations. Looking closer at the first equation of this set, the different contributions are in words:

$$\begin{bmatrix} \text{Rate of increase} \\ \text{of } u \text{ of a} \\ \text{fluid element} \end{bmatrix} + \begin{bmatrix} \text{Net rate of flow} \\ \text{of } u \text{ out of fluid} \\ \text{element (convection)} \end{bmatrix} = \begin{bmatrix} \text{Rate of increase} \\ \text{of } u \text{ due to} \\ \text{diffusion} \end{bmatrix} + \begin{bmatrix} \text{Rate of increase} \\ \text{of } u \text{ due to} \\ \text{sources} \end{bmatrix},$$

which means

$$\underbrace{\frac{\partial(\rho\boldsymbol{u})}{\partial t}}_{\substack{\text{rate of} \\ \text{change} \\ \text{term}}} + \underbrace{\rho\boldsymbol{u}\cdot\nabla\boldsymbol{u}}_{\substack{\text{convection} \\ \text{term}}} = \underbrace{-\nabla p + \nabla\cdot\left[\mu\left(\nabla\boldsymbol{u}+(\nabla\boldsymbol{u})^T\right)-\frac{2}{3}\mu\left(\nabla\cdot\boldsymbol{u}\right)\mathbf{I}\right]}_{\substack{\text{diffusion} \\ \text{term}}} + \underbrace{\rho\boldsymbol{b}}_{\substack{\text{source} \\ \text{term}}}.$$

Equations of that type are called transport equations of the variable u or convection-diffusion equations.

If the influence of the compressibility of the fluid flow is small, the fluid's density remains constant, hence $\frac{\partial\rho}{\partial t}\approx 0$. In cases with small density change this change is sometimes neglected to simplify equation (2.24) to the set of Navier Stokes Equations for incompressible, isothermal flow of Newtonian fluids:

$$\rho\frac{\partial\boldsymbol{u}}{\partial t} + \rho\boldsymbol{u}\cdot\nabla\boldsymbol{u} = -\nabla p + \nabla\cdot\left[\mu\left(\nabla\boldsymbol{u}+(\nabla\boldsymbol{u})^T\right)\right] + \rho\boldsymbol{b}$$
$$\nabla\cdot\boldsymbol{u} = 0. \tag{2.25}$$

A stationary solution is demanded, if not the time dependent behavior of the fluid motion is of interest, but the flow pattern, which is established in a certain setup under constant conditions. Hence, there are no variations with time, changing equation (2.24) to the set of stationary Navier Stokes Equations for compressible, isothermal flow of Newtonian fluids:

$$\rho\boldsymbol{u}\cdot\nabla\boldsymbol{u} = -\nabla p + \nabla\cdot\left[\mu\left(\nabla\boldsymbol{u}+(\nabla\boldsymbol{u})^T\right)-\frac{2}{3}\mu\left(\nabla\cdot\boldsymbol{u}\right)\mathbf{I}\right] + \rho\boldsymbol{b}$$
$$\nabla\cdot(\rho\boldsymbol{u}) = 0, \tag{2.26}$$

and with the assumption of incompressible flow the set of stationary Navier Stokes Equations for incompressible, isothermal flow of Newtonian fluids is given by

$$\rho\boldsymbol{u}\cdot\nabla\boldsymbol{u} = -\nabla p + \nabla\cdot\left[\mu\left(\nabla\boldsymbol{u}+(\nabla\boldsymbol{u})^T\right)\right] + \rho\boldsymbol{b}$$
$$\nabla\cdot\boldsymbol{u} = 0. \tag{2.27}$$

In flows very far away from solid walls, viscosity effects are often very small and are therefore neglected, so the stress tensor reduces to $T = -p\boldsymbol{I}$, compare (2.20). The resulting system is then called Euler equations and the flow is named *inviscid* flow and *viscous* flow in the contrary case.

Depending on the problem one of the presented forms of the Navier Stokes Equations can be used to simulate a fluid's behavior, but additional to these partial differential equations boundary conditions have to be defined. To begin, a qualitative distinction of the Navier Stokes Equations in the categories *elliptic*, *parabolic* or *hyperbolic* is given, which is dependent on the flow being steady or non-stationary, compressible or incompressible and viscous or inviscid. As already mentioned this distinction is only complete for linear second order equations in two independent variables, which is not the case for the Navier Stokes Equations, which are non-linear second order partial differential equations with four independent variables (one for the velocity in each spatial direction and the pressure). Xun [78] presented a classification of the Navier Stokes Equations based on weakly continuous surfaces. Ferziger and Perić [27] motivated a distinction qualitatively, that is summed up in the following:

Hyperbolic Flow
: In hyperbolic flows information propagates at finite speed in two sets of directions, compare figure 2.1. In an initial point a condition has to be given for each of the two characteristics, hence two boundary conditions have to be applied on every boundary. Inviscid compressible unsteady flows show this behavior, for steady flows, it depends on the flow velocity. In the supersonic case the flow is hyperbolic whereas elliptic in the subsonic case.

Parabolic Flow
: In parabolic flows transported information only propagates downstream, the definition of one boundary condition is sufficient. Unsteady flow shows this behavior except in the compressible inviscid case.

Elliptic Flow
: If flow has a recirculation area, information may travel upstream as well as downstream, the flow becomes elliptic then. One condition at every boundary is needed and the boundary has to be closed. Steady flows except the supersonic inviscid compressible flow show all elliptic character.

In table 2.1 the different classifications of the flow behavior are summarized.

Table 2.1: Classification of fluid flow in the classes that describe partial differential equations.

<table>
<tr><td rowspan="6">steady</td><td rowspan="2">incompressible</td><td>viscous</td><td rowspan="2"></td><td rowspan="5">elliptic</td></tr>
<tr><td>inviscid</td></tr>
<tr><td rowspan="4">compressible</td><td rowspan="2">viscous</td><td>subsonic</td></tr>
<tr><td>supersonic</td></tr>
<tr><td rowspan="2">inviscid</td><td>subsonic</td></tr>
<tr><td>supersonic</td><td>hyperbolic</td></tr>
<tr><td rowspan="6">unsteady</td><td rowspan="2">incompressible</td><td>viscous</td><td rowspan="2"></td><td rowspan="4">parabolic</td></tr>
<tr><td>inviscid</td></tr>
<tr><td rowspan="4">compressible</td><td rowspan="2">viscous</td><td>subsonic</td></tr>
<tr><td>supersonic</td></tr>
<tr><td rowspan="2">inviscid</td><td>subsonic</td><td rowspan="2">hyperbolic</td></tr>
<tr><td>supersonic</td></tr>
</table>

Turbulent Flow

Flow phenomena are distinguished in either laminar or turbulent flow. Laminar fluid motions are characterized by a high rate of regularity. The flow consists of individual slices flowing side by side without mixing, except diffusion in the microscope area by Brownian motion. Turbulent flow is characterized by the arise of vorticity and random motions crosswise to the direction of flow. Macroscopic motion energy is transformed to microscopic energy (heat) this process is called *dissipation*. In general flow is laminar in low velocities. By increase of the velocity the fluid field changes and fade to turbulent flow at a critical point.

Turbulence develops as a result of instabilities in the laminar flow, mathematical spoken it arises from interaction of the Navier Stokes Equation's nonlinear inertial terms and viscous terms. Physically spoken it arises from the interaction between motion fluctuations of different wavelength and directions. The motion is spread over a wide range of wavelength by vortex stretching, by what the turbulence gains energy. Larger-scale turbulent motion carries most of the energy and triggers enhanced diffusivity and attending stresses.

The dimensionless Reynolds number is a measure for the property of a flow to be turbulent or laminar. It sets the inertial forces in relation to the viscous forces, so that for a high Reynolds number the inertial forces are dominant. With L describing the characteristic length of a flow and ν denoting the kinematic viscosity and u the velocity magnitude, the Reynolds number is given by

$$\mathrm{Re} = \frac{\rho u L}{\mu} = \frac{u L}{\nu}. \tag{2.28}$$

In the circular pipe flow the characteristic length is the same as the pipe's diameter. For non-circular pipes the hydraulic diameter is used as characteristic length, it is defined as

$$D_H = \frac{4A}{P}, \tag{2.29}$$

where A is the cross sectional area of the pipe and P its wetted perimeter [71]. Fluid flow is laminar at "low" Reynolds numbers and becomes turbulent with rising Reynolds number. The point of inflection is called the critical Reynolds number. But the definition of that critical point is not trivial and problem dependent. For flow in long straight-lined pipes O. Reynold determined a critical Reynolds number of about 2300. But he himself estimated that the critical point of transition varies with the level of disturbance of the fluid flow [71]. R. Kerswell reported experimentally proven inflection points for this setup in the range of $1760 < \mathrm{Re} < 2300$ [41]. Often the area $2300 < \mathrm{Re} < 4000$ is seen as the transition area, where the change from laminar to turbulent flow takes place [76].

Figure 2.2 illustrates the transition from laminar to turbulent flow on a solid wall. The flow profile in the laminar region is hyperbolic, whereas the profile in the turbulent region is flattened further away from the wall, because of the appearance of vorticity and with that velocity components in the crosswise direction, as well as dissipation. The turbulent profile can be subdivided in four regimes:

- *viscous sublayer*: Near the wall the flow is linear with distance of the wall and laminar.

- *buffer layer*: After the viscous sublayer the transition to turbulent flow occurs.

- *log–law region*: In the turbulent region the flow shows at first a logarithmic profile with distance to the wall.

- *free stream region*: Then the flow becomes a free stream.

The viscous sublayer and the buffer region are quite small, the log–law region extends at about a hundred times the both first layers together. Although turbulent flow is of high research interest within the last decades, it is still a challenging task to rightly predict turbulent flow phenomena. Turbulence is a result of the instability of the laminar flow and is characterized by motion on widespread wavelength. Even the smallest eddies contribute to the turbulent flow field. As a result for the simulation of turbulent flow the resolution of all contributing scales is necessary. A resolution of all scales would require a very fine spatial discretization, which is in most cases not

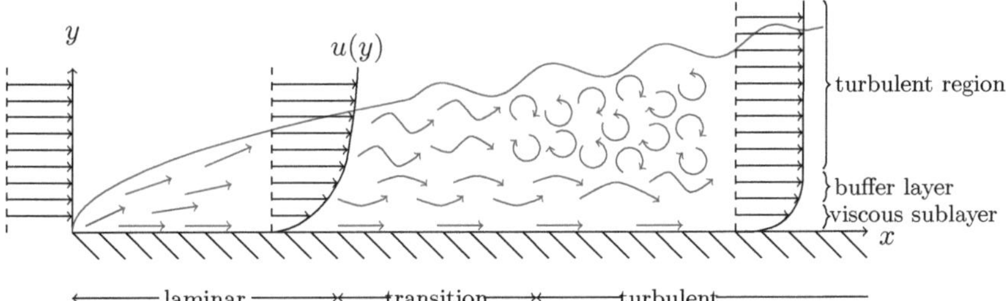

Figure 2.2: Visualization of the transition from laminar to turbulent flow at a solid boundary and the development of the characteristic boundary layers. After [75].

applicable due to computational costs. In [28] an estimate is given, that the number of needed points in a spatial discretization scales with the Reynolds number by $Re^{\frac{9}{4}}$, which means even for a low turbulent Reynolds number like 2000 a spatial grid with $2.675 \cdot 10^7$ nodes would be necessary, which is in general not realizable because of computational costs.

Some techniques have been developed to describe turbulent flow with less computational costs, by introducing some approximations. In general those are divided into Large eddy simulations and averaged Navier Stokes Equations. Large Eddy simulations use a spatial discretization that only resolves the largest eddies, the contribution of smaller eddies is modeled. Within this work the second type the averaged Navier Stokes Equations are used and therefore explained in more detail in the following.

The averaged Navier Stokes Equations are based on a statistical approach, which Reynolds introduced in 1895. The idea is to solve the governing equations for the mean velocity of the flow and neglecting the turbulent fluctuations by averaging over time. The flow is described by a sum of its mean parts $U_i(\boldsymbol{x})$ and its fluctuating parts $u_i'(\boldsymbol{x})$:

$$u_i(\boldsymbol{x}, t) = U_i(\boldsymbol{x}) + u_i'(\boldsymbol{x}, t), \tag{2.30}$$

with the mean velocity averaged over time

$$U_i(x) = \lim_{T \to \infty} \frac{1}{T} \int_t^{t+T} u_i(\boldsymbol{x}, t) \mathrm{d}t, \tag{2.31}$$

which is illustrated in figure 2.3. Let T_1 denote the maximum period of the turbulent fluctuation. In practice it is sufficient to chose a time $T >> T_1$ for averaging instead of $T \to \infty$. In the case of instationary flow equations (2.30) and (2.31) are replaced by

$$u_i(\boldsymbol{x}, t) = U_i(\boldsymbol{x}, t) + u_i'(\boldsymbol{x}, t) \tag{2.32}$$

and

$$U_i(\boldsymbol{x}, t) = \frac{1}{T} \int_t^{t+T} u_i(\boldsymbol{x}, t) \mathrm{d}t, \quad T_1 << T << T_2, \tag{2.33}$$

where T_2 is a time scale characteristic of the flow variations of the instationary flow. That indicates that there have to be several orders of magnitude distance between times T_1 and T_2, if that is not the case the method is not applicable.

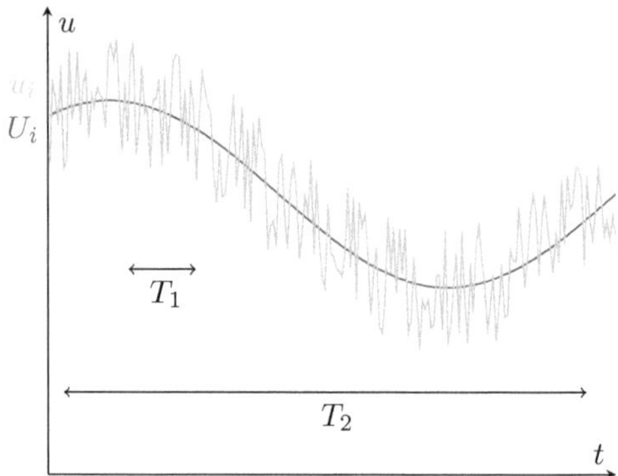

Figure 2.3: Time averaging eliminates the turbulent fluctuations of the velocity.

The Navier Stokes Equations are averaged over time, for simplicity reasons the incompressible Navier Stokes Equations (2.25) are regarded in the following. Let a bar over a variable denote the time average of the variable and P is the time averaged pressure: $\bar{p} = P$, then the averaged quantities are given by $\bar{u} = \bar{U} = U$ and

$$\frac{\overline{\partial u}}{\partial t} \approx \frac{\partial U}{\partial t} \quad \text{for } |u_i| << |U_i|. \tag{2.34}$$

The approximation of the derivative of the velocity with respect to time demands that the fluctuating part is small in relation to the mean velocity.

Regarding the time average over the product of two quantities ψ and ϕ, which are composed of a mean (Ψ, resp. Φ) and a fluctuating part (ψ', resp. ϕ'), correlations arise:

$$\overline{\psi\phi} = \overline{(\psi + \psi')(\phi + \phi')} = \overline{\Psi\Phi + \Psi\phi' + \Phi\psi' + \phi'\psi'} = \Psi\Phi + \overline{\psi'\phi'}. \tag{2.35}$$

The time average of the fluctuating part is zero and therefore the product of it with a mean value as well. But it is not known whether the product of the two fluctuating parts is zero or not. The quantities ϕ' and ψ' are said to be correlated for $\overline{\phi'\psi'} \neq 0$ and uncorrelated in the contrary case. For the time averaging of the incompressible Navier Stokes Equations, this is important by averaging the term $u \cdot \nabla u$, which then produces a correlation part. The time average of the incompressible Navier Stokes Equations, which are then called Reynolds Averaged Navier Stokes (RANS) Equations for incompressible flow are given by

$$\rho\frac{\partial U}{\partial t} + \rho U \cdot \nabla U + \nabla \cdot (\overline{\rho u' \otimes u'}) = -\nabla P + \nabla \cdot \mu(\nabla U + (\nabla U)^T) + \rho b \tag{2.36}$$

$$\frac{\partial U}{\partial t} = 0, \tag{2.37}$$

where $\otimes$ denotes the outer vector product. These equations are the same as the original incompressible Navier Stokes Equations with u replaced by the mean velocity U but with the additional term $\tau = -\overline{\rho u' \times u'}$, which is known as Reynolds stresses. Reynolds averaging produces 6 new unknowns in the governing equations, one Reynolds stress for each combination of the three spatial components, but it does not produce any more equations, leading to a closure problem. This is the starting point for the turbulence models. They introduce additional partial differential equations to the RANS equations with independent variables, which describe the turbulence of the flow and thereby close the system. The two most used turbulence models

$k - \epsilon$ model and $k - \omega$ model are presented within this context. More turbulence models can be found for example in [76]. One property of turbulent flow is the turbulent kinetic energy per unit mass k defined by

$$k = \frac{1}{2}(\overline{u_1'^2} + \overline{u_2'^2} + \overline{u_3'^2}). \tag{2.38}$$

The idea of the mentioned turbulence models is to add a partial differential equation to the system, which models the transport of the kinetic energy. The derivation of this transport equation is quite complex, it is explained in detail in [76]. The basic idea is to take moments of the Navier Stokes Equation by multiplying it with fluctuating velocity components and time average the product. In doing so a partial differential equation is derived describing the behavior of the Reynolds stresses. This equation is called Reynolds-Stress equation or Reynolds-Stress Transport equation. By identifying that $-2k/\rho$ is the trace of the Reynolds stresses τ, the transport equation of the turbulent kinetic energy can be derived by regarding the trace of the Reynolds-Stress equation. The k transport equation for incompressible flow reads as

$$\frac{\partial k}{\partial t} + \underbrace{\boldsymbol{U} \cdot \nabla k}_{\text{convection}} = \underbrace{\boldsymbol{\tau} \nabla \cdot \boldsymbol{U}}_{\text{production}} - \epsilon + \nabla \cdot \left[\underbrace{\nu \nabla k}_{\substack{\text{molecular} \\ \text{diffusion}}} \underbrace{- \frac{1}{2}\overline{\boldsymbol{U}'(\boldsymbol{U}' \otimes \boldsymbol{U}')}}_{\substack{\text{turbulent} \\ \text{transport}}} \underbrace{- \frac{1}{\rho}\overline{p'\boldsymbol{U}'}}_{\substack{\text{Pressure} \\ \text{diffusion}}} \right], \tag{2.39}$$

with the dissipation per unit mass

$$\epsilon = \nu \overline{\nabla \boldsymbol{U}' \cdot \nabla \boldsymbol{U}'}, \tag{2.40}$$

which is the rate of turbulent kinetic energy being transformed into thermal internal energy. The unsteady term and the convection term on the left hand side describe the rate of change of k following a fluid particle. The rate at which kinetic energy is transferred from the mean flow to turbulence is the production. The molecular diffusion represents diffusion of turbulent kinetic energy resulting from fluid's natural molecular transport processes. The rate at which kinetic energy is transported through the fluid by turbulent fluctuations is represented by the turbulent transport term and the turbulent transport resulting from correlation of pressure and velocity fluctuations is determined by the pressure diffusion. It should be remarked, that the k transport equation (2.39) is still exact. Based on this the modeling process starts. Whereas the unsteady term, the convection and the molecular diffusion are exact, the production, dissipation, pressure diffusion and turbulent transport terms involve unknown correlations. Hence, to close the system it is necessary to model the Reynolds stresses, the dissipation, the turbulent transport and the pressure diffusion. At first the Boussinesq approximation is applied, which states, that the Reynolds stresses can be approximated with [76]

$$\tau = 2\nu_T \boldsymbol{S} - \frac{2}{3}k\boldsymbol{I}, \tag{2.41}$$

where $\boldsymbol{I}$ is the identity matrix, the strain-rate tensor is given by

$$[S]_{ij} = \frac{1}{2}\left[\frac{\partial U_i}{\partial x_j} + \frac{\partial U_j}{\partial x_i}\right] \tag{2.42}$$

and ν_T is a component called *eddy viscosity*. Secondly an approximation is introduced, which groups the turbulent transport and the pressure diffusion and postulates, that the sum of them behaves as a gradient-transport process:

$$\frac{1}{2}\overline{\boldsymbol{U}'(\boldsymbol{U}' \otimes \boldsymbol{U}')} + \frac{1}{\rho}\overline{p'\boldsymbol{U}'} = -\frac{\nu_T}{\sigma_k}\nabla k, \tag{2.43}$$

where σ_k is a closure constant, which has to be determined experimentally. Still remaining is the definition of the eddy viscosity or equivalent the turbulent viscosity given by

$$\mu_T = \nu_T \rho \tag{2.44}$$

and the dissipation ϵ has to be modeled. The approaches differ from each other in the mentioned turbulence models.

$k - \omega$ model:

The $k - \omega$ turbulence model was first proposed by Kolmogorov in 1942 [43]. Despite the modeling of the turbulent kinetic energy, he used the dissipation per unit turbulence kinetic energy, also called specific dissipation rate, ω as second parameter with unit $[\omega] = t^{-1}$. The connection to the dissipation per unit mass ϵ is given by ω being somewhat like the ratio of ϵ to k despite additional constants. It is not reported how Kolmogorov arrived at his model equations, Wilcox [76] imagined, that Kolmogorov may have made a dimensional analysis resembling:

- it is plausible that $\nu_T \propto k$
- dimension of ν_T is (length)^2/(time) and that of k is (length)^2/(time)^2
- hence $\nu_t k^{-1}$ has dimensions (length)^2/(time)^3
- therefore ϵk^{-1} has dimensions (time)$^{-1}$
- the equations can be closed by introducing a variable with dimension (time)$^{-1}$.

Additionally to the dimensional analysis Wilcox assumed that Kolmogorov may have performed physical reasoning that a fluid property is affected by the physical processes of unsteadiness, convection, diffusion, dissipation, dispersion and production. Within this context the $k - \omega$ turbulence model is used with modifications by Wilcox [76] in the following form:

turbulent kinetic energy

$$\rho \frac{\partial k}{\partial t} + \rho \boldsymbol{U} \cdot \nabla k = P_k - \rho \beta^* k \omega + \nabla \cdot [(\mu + \sigma^* \mu_T) \nabla k] \tag{2.45}$$

specific dissipation rate

$$\rho \frac{\partial \omega}{\partial t} + \rho \boldsymbol{U} \cdot \nabla \omega = \alpha \frac{\omega}{k} P_k - \rho \beta \omega^2 + \nabla \cdot [(\mu + \sigma \mu_T) \nabla \omega] \tag{2.46}$$

with the

production term

$$P_k = \mu_T \left[\nabla \boldsymbol{U} : (\nabla \boldsymbol{U} + (\nabla \boldsymbol{U})^T) - \frac{2}{3}(\nabla \cdot \boldsymbol{U})^2 \right] - \frac{2}{3}\rho k \nabla \cdot \boldsymbol{U} \tag{2.47}$$

where the colon operator takes the product of the components as $[a : b]_{ij} = a_{ij} b_{ij}$. And it is given the

turbulent viscosity

$$\mu_T = \rho \frac{k}{\omega} \tag{2.48}$$

and the

closure coefficients

$$\alpha = \frac{13}{25} \quad \beta = \beta_0 f_\beta \quad \beta^* = \beta_0^* f_{\beta*} \quad \sigma = \frac{1}{2} \quad \sigma^* = \frac{1}{2} \tag{2.49}$$

$$\beta_0 = \frac{13}{125} \quad f_\beta = \frac{1 + 70\mathcal{X}_\omega}{1 + 80\mathcal{X}_\omega} \quad \mathcal{X}_\omega = \left| \frac{\boldsymbol{\Omega}_{ij}\boldsymbol{\Omega}_{jk}\boldsymbol{S}ki}{(\beta_0^*\omega)^3} \right| \tag{2.50}$$

$$\beta_0^* = \frac{9}{100} \quad f_{\beta*} = \begin{cases} 1 & \mathcal{X}_k \le 0 \\ \frac{1+680\mathcal{X}_k^2}{1+400\mathcal{X}_k^2} & \mathcal{X}_k > 0 \end{cases} \quad \mathcal{X}_k = \frac{1}{\omega^3}(\nabla k \cdot \nabla \omega), \tag{2.51}$$

where Einstein's sum convention[2] is used to describe $\mathcal{X}_\omega$. Where $\boldsymbol{S}$ is the strain rate tensor defined in (2.42) and $\boldsymbol{\Omega}$ is the mean-rotation tensor

$$[\Omega]_{ij} = \frac{1}{2}\left[\frac{\partial U_i}{\partial x_j} - \frac{\partial U_j}{\partial x_i}\right]. \tag{2.52}$$

Closure coefficients as well as closure approximations are thereby introduced using experimental results. So they are fitted to resemble the measured behavior.

The transport equation can not be implemented as they are described, because nothing prevents division by zero. Therefore a realizability constant is included and limits for the turbulent viscosity. Which is explained in more detail in the description of the $k - \epsilon$ model. The flow near solid walls is very different to the free stream region as indicated in figure 2.2. The assumptions to derive the closure approximations and the governing equations are not valid anymore in the near-wall regions. To deal with this problem so called wall functions are applied. Wall functions make use of one of the most famous empirically determined relations of the behavior of turbulent flow near solid boundaries. As figure 2.2 indicates the flow pattern near solid walls has a logarithmic shape for turbulent flows. Effects of fluid's inertia and pressure gradients are observed to be small near the surface, the remaining and determining effects are the rate at which momentum is transferred to the surface and the molecular diffusion of momentum. The flow field near walls is therefore assumed to be describable with this two effects in an logarithmic function with respect to the wall distance [76]. Let therefore y denote the distance to the nearest surface. A velocity scale representative for the velocity near the surface is introduced: the friction velocity

$$u_\tau = \sqrt{\frac{\tau_w}{\rho}}, \tag{2.53}$$

where τ_w is the surface shear stress. With the friction velocity also a length scale ν/u_τ is determined. The variation of the velocity with respect to the distance to the surface should depend on those scales and y. With dimensional analysis this yields

$$\frac{\partial \boldsymbol{U}}{\partial y} = \frac{u_\tau}{y} F\left(\frac{u_\tau y}{\nu}\right). \tag{2.54}$$

Experimentally it is determined that

$$\lim_{u_\tau y/\nu \to \infty} F\left(\frac{u_\tau y}{\nu}\right) \to \frac{1}{\kappa}, \tag{2.55}$$

---

[2] Einstein's sum convention for matrices $\boldsymbol{A}$, $\boldsymbol{B}$ is a notation abbreviation, where writing same indices is meant to take the sum over the elements with same index: $\boldsymbol{A}_{ij}\boldsymbol{B}_{jk} := \boldsymbol{C}$ with $c_{ik} = \sum_j a_{ij}b_{jk}$

where $\kappa = 0.41$ is Karman's constant. Integrating over y yields the famous *law of the wall* [76]

$$\frac{U}{u_\tau} = \frac{1}{\kappa} \ln \frac{u_\tau y}{\nu} + C, \tag{2.56}$$

where C is an integration constant, indicated by measurements it follows that $C \approx 5$. This flow pattern near surfaces is adjusted in flow simulations by restricting the computational domain for the described transport equations to an area with a distance δ_w to the wall, which is chosen in the way that the wall distance in viscous units defined by

$$\delta_w^+ = \rho u_\tau \frac{\delta_w}{\mu} \tag{2.57}$$

with the friction velocity computed by

$$u_\tau = \beta_0^{*\frac{1}{4}} \sqrt{k} \tag{2.58}$$

becomes 11.06, which corresponds to the distance in viscous units, where the logarithmic layer to some extend would meet the viscous sublayer, if there would not be the buffer layer in between. From the law of the wall it follows that

$$u_\tau = \frac{|U|}{\kappa^{-1} \ln \delta_w + B}, \tag{2.59}$$

with $B \approx 5.2$ empirically determined. This relation is used to prescribe the velocity with a shear stress condition

$$\boldsymbol{n} \cdot \boldsymbol{\sigma} - (\boldsymbol{n} \cdot \boldsymbol{\sigma} \cdot \boldsymbol{n})\boldsymbol{n} = -\rho u_\tau \frac{\boldsymbol{U}}{|\boldsymbol{U}|} \max(\beta_0^* \sqrt{k}, u_\tau), \tag{2.60}$$

and also a non-penetration condition

$$\boldsymbol{U} \cdot \boldsymbol{n} = 0. \tag{2.61}$$

The turbulent kinetic energy is prescribed with a homogeneous Neumann's condition

$$\boldsymbol{n} \cdot \nabla k = 0. \tag{2.62}$$

And it is assumed that the following condition is valid

$$\omega = \frac{\rho k}{\kappa \delta_w^+ \mu}. \tag{2.63}$$

Using this wall function conditions in the area of the boundary layer instead of the model equations leads to a better near wall flow prediction.

$k - \epsilon$ model:

In the $k - \epsilon$ model also a transport equation of the turbulent kinematic energy is used. The second governing equation is a partial differential equation of the dissipation ϵ. Therefore again moments of the Navier Stokes Equations are taken to derive an exact equation for the transport of ϵ. But those equation is far more complex than the one for k and involves more unknowns, which have to be modeled using again dimensional analysis and physical reasoning as well as closure coefficients and approximations. The idea of $k - \epsilon$ model was firstly used by Chou [15], Davidov [20] and Harlow and Nakayama [33]. The model has its wide spread use with the changes of the closure coefficients by Launder and Sharma [45], which is in general referred to as the *Standard $k - \epsilon$* model. The model equations used are as follows

turbulent kinetic energy

$$\rho\frac{\partial k}{\partial t} + \rho\boldsymbol{U} \cdot \nabla k = \nabla \cdot \left[(\mu + \frac{\mu_T}{\sigma_k})\nabla k\right] + P_k - \rho\epsilon, \tag{2.64}$$

where the production term P_k is defined in (2.47).

dissipation rate

$$\rho\frac{\partial \epsilon}{\partial t} + \rho\boldsymbol{U} \cdot \nabla \epsilon = \nabla \cdot \left[(\mu + \frac{\mu_T}{\sigma_\epsilon})\nabla \epsilon\right] + C_{\epsilon 1}\frac{\epsilon}{k}P_k - C_{\epsilon 2}\rho\frac{\epsilon^2}{k} \tag{2.65}$$

turbulent viscosity

$$\mu_T = \rho C_\mu \frac{k^2}{\epsilon} \tag{2.66}$$

With the

closure coefficients

$$C_\mu = 0.09 \quad C_{\epsilon 1} = 1.44 \quad C_{\epsilon 2} = 1.92$$
$$\sigma_k = 1.0 \quad \sigma_\epsilon = 1.3 \tag{2.67}$$

Some remarks on necessary changes to the turbulence model equations for the implementation are given in the following:
A linearization variable $\gamma = \frac{\epsilon}{k}$ is introduced to decouple the turbulent kinetic energy and dissipation equation, leading to

$$\rho\frac{\partial k}{\partial t} + \rho\boldsymbol{U} \cdot \nabla k = \nabla \cdot \left[(\mu + \frac{\mu_T}{\sigma_k})\nabla k\right] + P_k - \rho\gamma k \tag{2.68}$$

$$\rho\frac{\partial \epsilon}{\partial t} + \rho\boldsymbol{U} \cdot \nabla \epsilon = \nabla \cdot \left[(\mu + \frac{\mu_T}{\sigma_\epsilon})\nabla \epsilon\right] + \gamma(C_{\epsilon 1}P_k - C_{\epsilon 2}\rho\epsilon). \tag{2.69}$$

The variable γ is updated in an iterative solution process by

$$\gamma = C_\mu \frac{k}{\rho\mu_T}. \tag{2.70}$$

μ_T is calculated by

$$\mu_T = \rho l_{\text{mix}}\sqrt{k}, \tag{2.71}$$

where l_{mix} is the mixing length

$$l_{\text{mix}} = \min\left(C_\mu \frac{k^{\frac{3}{2}}}{\epsilon}, l_+\right) \tag{2.72}$$

where the upper bound is the mixing length limit l_+, which is the maximal size of an eddy, e.g. the domain size. This demand guarantees that no division by zero is performed. The mixing length is secondly subjected to a realizability constraint:

$$l_+ \leq \frac{1}{\sqrt{6}}\frac{\sqrt{k}}{\sqrt{\sum\limits_{i,j} s_{ij}s_{ij}}} = l_r. \tag{2.73}$$

This constraint is necessary, because the Reynolds stresses should be nonnegative, but this is not guaranteed with using only equation (2.48). With the two mentioned constrictions on the mixing length and the decoupling of the turbulent kinetic energy equation and the dissipation equation it is achieved to preclude division by zero and to have bounded nonnegative coefficients without manipulating the values of k and ϵ. More information on that can be found in [44].

The $k - \omega$ model uses the same implementation strategy, the mixing length is in that case bounded by

$$l_{\mathrm{mix}} = \min\left(\frac{\sqrt{k}}{\omega}, l_+, l_r\right). \tag{2.74}$$

The $k - \epsilon$ model also uses wall functions in the same manner as explained for the $k - \omega$ model, but the constant β_0^* is replaced by C_μ. It is assumed that dissipation and production are in equilibrium in the near wall layer yielding the condition

$$\epsilon = \frac{C_\mu^{\frac{3}{4}} k^{\frac{3}{2}}}{k} \kappa \delta_w. \tag{2.75}$$

Within the wide area of turbulence models, the $k - \epsilon$ and the $k - \omega$ model are the most used models in the past decades. But turbulence models always rely on some assumptions and are calibrated with experimental data and if a model fits for one experimental setup it is not sure if it fits for another one. The $k - \epsilon$ model relies on the assumptions of a high Reynolds number and dissipation and production being in equilibrium within the boundary layer. It is known, that it performs not very well in flow with adverse pressure gradient by underestimating spatial extensions of recirculation zones [76] and the agreement with experimental data of rotating flows is not quite good [23]. But the $k - \epsilon$ model has a good convergence rate and is very popular because of its computational efficiency. The $k - \omega$ model performs in many cases better than the $k - \epsilon$ model [23]. But it is very sensitive to free stream values of ω [76] and it is as well as the $k - \epsilon$ model designed for high Reynolds number flows and for fully developed turbulent flow, e.g. the closure coefficients are estimated using experimental data of fully developed turbulent flow, which makes it difficult to apply turbulence models in the transitional area.

2.2.2 Finite Element Method

The Finite Element Method (FEM) is a numerical tool delivering approximated solutions to partial differential equations. The basic idea is to introduce a spatial discretization in a finite set of elements K and nodes of the regarded area Ω on which the PDE shall be solved. This partitioning of Ω is called triangulation T with $T = \{K\}$. Usually those elements are simplex or cuboid structures. Figure 2.4 shows exemplary a triangular discretization of a two dimensional Ω. A triangulation is regular if it fulfills three requirements:

Definition 2.4 (valid triangulation) *A triangulation T is regular if*

(i) $\Omega = \bigcup_{K \in T} K$

(ii) $K_i \backslash \partial K_i \cap K_j \backslash \partial K_j = \emptyset \ \forall K_i, K_j \in T, K_i \neq K_j$

(iii) $\forall K_i \in T$: *every part of the boundary ∂K_i is either part of $\partial \Omega$ or part of the boundary ∂K_j of another element $K_j \in T, K_i \neq K_j$.*

In the application also triangulations are in usage which not exactly match all three requirements like figure 2.4, where the curved boundary of Ω is approximated by linear boundaries of the triangles. This approximation can be circumvented by using curved elements as can be found for example in [68]. After Ciarlet [16] a finite element can be defined as follows:

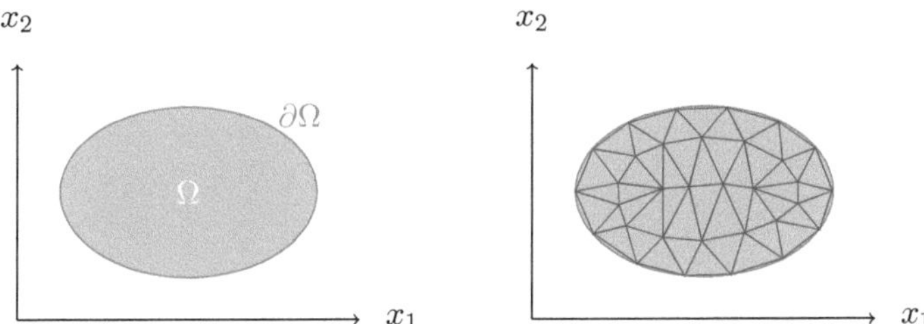

Figure 2.4: The Finite Element Method performs a spatial discretization on the regarded area Ω resulting in a finite set of elements and nodes.

Definition 2.5 (finite element) *A d-dimensional finite element is a triple $(K, P^{(K)}, N^{(K)})$ where K is a closed bounded subset of R^d with piecewise smooth boundary, $P^{(K)}$ is a finite-dimensional vector space defined over K, and $N^{(K)}$ is the basis of the space that contains all linear mappings $\phi : P^{(K)} \to K$, called the* dual space $P^{(K)^*}$. $P^{(K)}$ *is called the* shape space. $N^{(K)}$ *are the node values, also called the* degrees of freedom.

Remark that these explanations are for only one dependent variable to solve, in this case the number of nodes and the degrees of freedom are the same, this is not the case, if more dependent variables are considered.

Having defined a triangulation consisting of elements $K_i \in T$, $i \in \{1, ..., n_K\}$ and a finite amount of nodes N_j , $j \in \{1, ..., n_N\}$ without spaces between adjacent element boundaries, the shape functions have to be defined. Generally these are polynomials. For simplicity reasons these basis functions are presented with an one dimensional example consisting of only two mesh elements $E_1 : \ 0 < x < 1$ and $E_2 : \ 1 < x < 2$. In usage of linear basis functions a one dimensional mesh element has got a node at the beginning of the line and one at the end, resulting in three nodes for the simple example, see figure 2.5(a). The basis function ϕ_j is now prescribed to equal one at the jth node and zero at other nodes. For the linear case, this demand results in

$$\phi_1(x) = \begin{cases} 1 - x & \text{, if } 0 \leq x < 1 \\ 0 & \text{, else} \end{cases} \tag{2.76}$$

and analogously for the other basis functions. In the case of quadratic basis functions, five nodes have to be regarded in the one dimensional example, see figure 2.5b, the quadratic basis function is given by

$$\phi_1 = \begin{cases} (1 - x)(1 - 2x) & \text{, if } 0 \leq x < 1 \\ 0 & \text{, else} \end{cases} . \tag{2.77}$$

The two element types presented here are special cases of Lagrange elements. Considering a positive integer k those elements have shape functions of polynomial type with a degree of k. The values of the nodes $U_j^{(k)}$ corresponding to one element K are used to define the basis functions. In the first example linear Lagrange elements with $k = 1$ are presented and in the second one quadratic elements with $k = 2$. There are some other element types like Hermitian

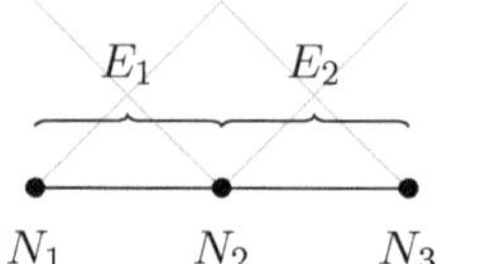

(a) Linear quadratic functions

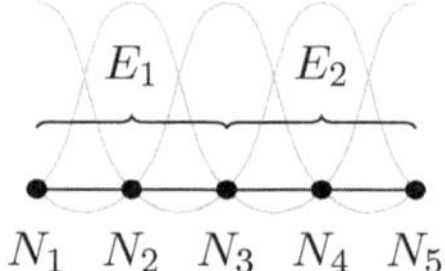

(b) Quadratic basis functions

Figure 2.5: One dimensional example of finite element mesh with two mesh elements and linear basis functions in (a) and quadratic basis functions in (b). The shape functions are indicated in blue.

elements, which use derivatives of u at the nodes to specify the basis functions. Other elements are not regarded within this context, because Lagrange elements are the most established ones, an overview of different two dimensional elements can be found for example in [9].

With the defined elements and belonging shape functions an approximation of the dependent variables u of the PDE are introduced which has the form

$$u(x) \approx u_l(\boldsymbol{U}) = \sum_{j=1}^{n_N} \phi_j(x)U_j, \tag{2.78}$$

where $\boldsymbol{U} = [U_j]_{j=1}^{n_N}$ are the values $U_j = u(N_j)$ at the node positions N_j and ϕ_j are the shape functions. By inserting this approximation in the PDE, it is transformed to a system of algebraic equations whose unknown variables are the finite set of values at the nodal positions. The following explanations are orientated at the implementation in the COMSOL© simulation tool, a more detailed description can be found in the corresponding manual [18].

The discretization of the Dirichlet's boundary conditions can be achieved by prescribing the values at the node positions

$$U_j = u_D(N_j) \quad \forall U_j \text{ on } \Gamma_D. \tag{2.79}$$

Therefore Dirichlet's boundary conditions can be summarized in a system of algebraic equations

$$\boldsymbol{M} = [M(U_i)]_{i=1}^{n_N} = \boldsymbol{0}, \tag{2.80}$$

where

$$M(U_i) = \begin{cases} U_i - u_D(N_i), & \text{if } N_i \in \Gamma_D \\ 0, & \text{else} \end{cases}. \tag{2.81}$$

The Neumann's boundary conditions are included in the weak form of the PDE. Consider the weak equation

$$0 = \int_\Omega W \, \mathrm{dA} - \int_{\partial\Omega} \tilde{u} h \lambda \, \mathrm{ds}. \tag{2.82}$$

The stationary solution is demanded. The space of test functions is chosen to be the same as the finite space, which is known as Galerkin's method, see for example [68]

$$\tilde{u}_j = \sum_{i=1}^{n_N} \phi_i \gamma_i, \quad j = 1 \ldots \dim(V), \ \gamma_i \in \mathbb{R}. \tag{2.83}$$

The test functions $\tilde{u}$ only occur in linear dependency and the weak form must hold for every test function in the chosen space - here the finite space, therefore it is sufficient to choose the basis functions as test functions

$$\tilde{u}_i = \phi_i, \quad i = 1 \ldots n_N \tag{2.84}$$

resulting in a system of equations, counting n_N functions, one for every i, as much as there are degrees of freedom. In the simplest case of only one dependent variable, there are as many equations as there are nodes in the mesh.

The integral

$$\int_{\partial \Omega} \phi_i \cdot h \lambda \mathrm{ds} \tag{2.85}$$

is approximated by a sum over all mesh elements, where the contribution of one element K is determined by a Riemann sum

$$\sum_j \phi_i(N_j^{(K)}) \cdot h(N_j^{(K)}) \lambda(N_j^{(K)}) w_j^{(K)} \tag{2.86}$$

where w_j is a weighting factor, which is the length of the appropriate part of the mesh element.

$$\left[\mathbf{\Lambda}^{(K)} \right]_j = \lambda(N_j^{(K)}) w_j^{(K)} \tag{2.87}$$

are the discretized Lagrange multipliers. The integral over Ω is approximated in the same manner. This results in an algebraic equation for every i forming together a system

$$0 = \boldsymbol{L} - \boldsymbol{N}\boldsymbol{\Lambda}, \tag{2.88}$$

where the ith row of $\boldsymbol{L}$ is

$$[\boldsymbol{L}]_i = \int_\Omega W \, \mathrm{dA} \tag{2.89}$$

evaluated for $\tilde{u} = \phi_i$. $\boldsymbol{\Lambda}$ is a vector of all discretized Lagrange multipliers and $\boldsymbol{N}$ is a matrix, where the ith row is a concatenation of the vectors

$$[\boldsymbol{N}]_i = \phi_i(N_j^{(K)}) \, h(N_j^{(K)}). \tag{2.90}$$

The finite space is spanned by the degrees of freedom $\boldsymbol{U}$, which means that the shape functions ϕ_i are functions of $\boldsymbol{U}$, hence the PDE (2.82) can be transformed to

$$0 = \boldsymbol{L}(\boldsymbol{U}) - \boldsymbol{N}(\boldsymbol{U})\boldsymbol{\Lambda} \tag{2.91}$$
$$0 = \boldsymbol{M}, \tag{2.92}$$

where $\boldsymbol{U}$ is the solution vector, which shall be solved for. For a time dependent problem the resulting algebraic system would look similar to

$$0 = \boldsymbol{L}(\boldsymbol{U}, \dot{\boldsymbol{U}}, \ddot{\boldsymbol{U}}, t) - \boldsymbol{N}(\boldsymbol{U}, t)\boldsymbol{\Lambda} \tag{2.93}$$
$$0 = \boldsymbol{M}(t). \tag{2.94}$$

For the solution of time dependent problems also a time discretization is needed, which is referred to in the next chapter.

Considering a nonlinear PDE as the Navier Stokes Equation the system of algebraic equation is also nonlinear and is alike to

$$\mathbf{0} = \boldsymbol{L}(\boldsymbol{U})\boldsymbol{U} - \boldsymbol{N}(\boldsymbol{U})\boldsymbol{\Lambda} \tag{2.95}$$

$$\mathbf{0} = \boldsymbol{M}. \tag{2.96}$$

In order to solve the discretized PDE a linearization of the algebraic system of equations is needed which is referred to in the following chapter.

2.2.3 Numerical Solution

Stabilization

Convection-diffusion equations are known to produce numerical difficulties if the convection part is dominant [37]. The momentum equation of the Navier Stokes Equations (2.24) can be transformed into a dimensionless form by normalizing the time with a reference time t_0, the velocity with the mean velocity magnitude U, the spatial coordinates with the length scale L and the pressure with ρU^2:

$$t^* = \frac{t}{t_0}, \quad x_i^* = \frac{x_i}{L}, \quad \boldsymbol{u}^* = \frac{\boldsymbol{u}}{U}, \quad p^* = \frac{p}{\rho U^2}. \tag{2.97}$$

The momentum equation becomes

$$\mathrm{St}\frac{\partial(\boldsymbol{u}^*)}{\partial t^*} + \boldsymbol{u}^* \cdot \nabla^*\boldsymbol{u}^* = -\nabla^*p + \nabla^* \cdot \frac{1}{\mathrm{Re}} \left[\left(\nabla^*\boldsymbol{u}^* + (\nabla^*\boldsymbol{u}^*)^T\right) - \frac{2}{3}\left(\nabla^* \cdot \boldsymbol{u}^*\right)\mathbf{I} \right] + \frac{L}{U^2}\boldsymbol{b}, \tag{2.98}$$

where $\nabla^* = [\frac{\partial}{\partial x_1^*}, \frac{\partial}{\partial x_2^*}, \frac{\partial}{\partial x_3^*}]^T$, and $\mathrm{St} = \frac{L}{Ut_0}$ is the Strouhal number. This shows that for high Reynolds numbers the contribution of the diffusion term is reduced and the convection term becomes dominant. Flows with high Reynolds numbers, turbulent flows, can produce numerical difficulties in the solution of the governing equations. The difficulties are a result of the solution possessing small regions with high gradients, which are not resolved by the mesh and therefore produce unwanted spurious, nonphysical oscillations in the numerical solution preventing numerical solvers from converging. Therefore stabilization techniques appropriate for convection-diffusion equations are needed. Those techniques are either

consistent
   if the solution of the non-stabilized equations also solves the stabilized equation,

inconsistent
   if the solution of the non-stabilized equation not necessarily solves the stabilized equation.

Inconsistent stabilization techniques have to be used with care, because they may introduce a systematical error.

One very established stabilization technique is the *Streamline Upwind Petrov Galerkin stabilization* (SUPG) developed by Brooks and Hughes [12]. The basic idea of this stabilization technique is to add artificial diffusion in the weak form of the convection-diffusion equation, which only acts in the streamline direction of the flow. This can be interpreted as modification of the test functions by applying the modification to all terms of the weak form, consistency is ensured. For a detailed description of the method see [12]. The additional diffusion reduces the dominance of the convection term, the solution becomes smooth and exact in smooth regions but it still can contain oscillations at sharp gradients. A second stabilization is often used to reduce this overshoots, called the *Crosswind Diffusion Stabilization*. Here again artificial diffusion is added to the weak form of the convection-diffusion equation, but this time orthogonal to the streamline direction which is the crosswind direction. The Crosswind Diffusion is a consistent stabilization technique, too. More information on Crosswind Diffusion and other Stabilization techniques can be found in [37]. By applying the two mentioned stabilization techniques numerical difficulties during the solving convection-diffusion equations like the Navier Stokes Equations can be reduced.

Time Discretization

If the problem to be solved is not a stationary but a time dependent one like (2.94), additionally to the spatial discretization a time discretization has to be performed. Within this case, the time discretization is performed after the spatial discretization, which is called the *method of lines*.
For simplicity reasons a spatial discretized system with only one time derivative is regarded:

$$0 = \boldsymbol{L}(\boldsymbol{U}, \dot{\boldsymbol{U}}, t) - \boldsymbol{N}(\boldsymbol{U}, t)\Lambda \tag{2.99}$$
$$0 = \boldsymbol{M}(t), \tag{2.100}$$

the second derivative can be included by applying the following differentiation scheme a second time.
Within the COMSOL$^{\copyright}$ implementation a variable time step, variable order, backward differentiation formula (BDF) is used in an algorithm called IDA, invented by the Lawrence Livermore National Laboratory [13], which is an enhancement of the DASPK algorithm by Hindmarsh et al. [35].
IDA is an iterative solving process, where the derivative of the solution at the nth time point t_n is described by a sum of the solutions at previous time steps

$$\sum_{i=0}^{q} \alpha_{n,i} \boldsymbol{U}_{n-i} = h_n \dot{\boldsymbol{U}}_n, \tag{2.101}$$

where $\boldsymbol{U}_j$, $\dot{\boldsymbol{U}}_j$, $j \in \{1, ..., n\}$ denotes the solution at the time t_j, $h_j = t_j - t_{j-1}$ is the time step size, which is variable for every iteration as well as the order q. The coefficients $\alpha_{i,n}$ can be determined by the order q and the knowledge of the step size's history. The solution in every time step can than be computed by solving

$$0 = \boldsymbol{L}\left(\boldsymbol{U}_n, h_n^{-1} \sum_{i=0}^{q} \alpha_{n,i} \boldsymbol{U}_{n-i}, t_n\right) - \boldsymbol{N}(\boldsymbol{U}_n, t_n)\Lambda \tag{2.102}$$

with a nonlinear solver, see the following section.
The choice of the variable step size and the order are performed with respect to local truncation error estimates, an exact description can be found in [13].

Nonlinear Solver

The nonlinear solver as it is used in COMSOL$^{\copyright}$ is a damped Newton method, comparable to the method presented in [22]. In the following the basic idea is given by the pseudocode algorithm. The input parameter are an initial guess to the solution $\boldsymbol{U}_0$, a lower bound to the damping factor

λ_{min}, a recovery damping factor λ_{rec}, a maximal number of iterations it_{max} and two tolerance limits tol_1 and tol_2. Let $f(\boldsymbol{U}) = 0$ denote the discretized system, that has to be solved, so that $\boldsymbol{U}$ is the solution vector and $F = f(\boldsymbol{U})$ is the residual vector, M is the number of nodes and N_j is the number of degrees of freedom of the node with number j. A double superscript index i, j denotes the ith degree of freedom belonging to the node with number j.

Data: $\boldsymbol{U}_0$, λ_{min}, λ_{rec}, it_{max}, tol_1, tol_2

Result: converged solution $\boldsymbol{U}_{k+1}$ or error if maximal number of iterations reached

Functions: $\mathrm{err}_1(\boldsymbol{U}, \boldsymbol{E}) = \sqrt{\dfrac{1}{M} \sum\limits_{j=1}^{M} \dfrac{1}{N_j} \sum\limits_{i=1}^{N_j} \left[\dfrac{|E_{i,j}|}{W_{i,j}} \right]^2}$;

$$\text{with } W_{i,j} = \max \left(|U_{i,j}|, 10^{-5} \cdot \dfrac{1}{N_j} \sum\limits_{i=1}^{N_j} |U_{i,j}| \right);$$

$$\mathrm{err}_2(\boldsymbol{U}) = \sqrt{\dfrac{1}{M} \sum\limits_{j=1}^{M} \dfrac{1}{N_j W_j} \sum\limits_{i=1}^{N_j} |F_{i,j}|^2 \cdot 1000};$$

$$\text{with } W_j = \sum\limits_{i=1}^{N_j} W_{i,j};$$

Initialization: $\boldsymbol{U}_{k+1} = \boldsymbol{U}_0, k = 0, e_{1_{k+1}} = \infty, e_{2_{k+1}} = \infty$;

while $k \leq it_{max}$ AND $\lambda \neq 1$ AND $e_{1_{k+1}} > tol_1$ AND $e_{2_{k+1}} > tol_2$ **do**

    $\boldsymbol{U}_k = \boldsymbol{U}_{k+1}$;

    $e_{1_{\mathrm{old}}} = 0, e_{1_{\mathrm{new}}} = \infty$;

    $k = k + 1$;

    SET $\lambda \in [\lambda_{\mathrm{min}}, 1]$;

    SOLVE $f'(\boldsymbol{U}_k)\partial \boldsymbol{U} = -f(\boldsymbol{U}_k)$ FOR $\partial \boldsymbol{U}$;

    while $e_{1_{new}} > e_{1_{old}}$ **do**

        $\boldsymbol{U}_{k+1} = \boldsymbol{U}_k + \lambda\, \partial \boldsymbol{U}$;

        Solve $f'(\boldsymbol{U}_{k+1})\boldsymbol{E} = -f(\boldsymbol{U}_k)$ FOR $\boldsymbol{E}$;

        $e_{\mathrm{new}} = \mathrm{err}_1(\boldsymbol{U}_{k+1}, \boldsymbol{E})$;

        REDUCE λ;

        if $\lambda < \lambda_{min}$ **then**

            $\boldsymbol{U}_{k+1} = \boldsymbol{U}_k + \lambda_{\mathrm{rec}}\, \partial \boldsymbol{U}$;

            $e_{1_{k+1}} = e_{\mathrm{new}}$;

            EXIT LOOP;

        end

    end

    $\boldsymbol{U}_{k+1} = \boldsymbol{U}_{\mathrm{new}}$;

    $e_{1_{k+1}} = e_{\mathrm{new}}$;

    $e_{2_{k+1}} = \mathrm{err}_2(\boldsymbol{U}_{k+1})$;

end

Algorithm 1: nonlinear damped Newton method

The nonlinear damped Newton solver requires a solution method for the linearized system $f'(\boldsymbol{U}_k)\partial \boldsymbol{U} = -f(\boldsymbol{U}_k)$. The linear system can be solved directly or iteratively, see the following section.

Linear solution process

The nonlinear damped Newton method derives a linearization of the governing equations, but still the linear system $f'(\boldsymbol{U}_k)\partial \boldsymbol{U} = -f(\boldsymbol{U}_k)$ has to be solved. Therefore a direct or an iterative solver can be used. The direct solver is more memory expensive than iterative solvers. In the following a direct solver PARDISO and an iterative solver GMRES are presented, which are used within the COMSOL© simulation environment.

PARDISO linear direct solver PARDISO is a high-performance and robust software, that is designed to efficiently solve linear systems with parallel computing and memory sharing [66]. The software is available at [65]. Given a linear system of equations $\boldsymbol{Ax} = \boldsymbol{b}$ with $\boldsymbol{A} \in \mathbb{R}^{N \times N}$, $\boldsymbol{x} \in \mathbb{R}^N$, $\boldsymbol{b} \in \mathbb{R}^N$ the idea of the direct solver PARDISO is to split the system matrix $\boldsymbol{A}$ into a factorization

$$\boldsymbol{A} = \boldsymbol{LU}, \tag{2.103}$$

where $\boldsymbol{L}$ is a lower triangular matrix and $\boldsymbol{U}$ is an upper triangular matrix. This is called LU-decomposition. The solution is then divided into two steps

$$\boldsymbol{Ly} = \boldsymbol{b} \tag{2.104}$$
$$\boldsymbol{Ux} = \boldsymbol{y} \tag{2.105}$$

The solution of both systems can easily be obtained by using forward substitution in the case of solving system 2.104:

for $m = 1 : N$ **do**
$\quad y_m = \frac{b_m - \sum_{i=1}^{m-1} l_{mi} y_i}{l_{mm}};$
end

with l_{ij} is the element of the matrix $\boldsymbol{L}$ in the ith row and the jth column, and backward substitution in the case of system 2.105:

for $m = N : 1$ **do**
$\quad x_m = \frac{y_m - \sum_{i=N}^{m+1} u_{mi} x_i}{u_{mm}};$
end

with u_{ij} is the element of the matrix $\boldsymbol{U}$ in the ith row and the jth column. Further details on the implementation can be found in [66].

GMRES linear iterative solver The GMRES (**G**eneral **M**inimal **RES**idual) linear solver was invented by Saad and Schultz in 1986 [64]. It is an iterative solver algorithm, that is robust and able to solve nonsymmetric problems. It is especially efficient for sparse matrix systems.
The GMRES algorithm is intended to solve a linear system $\boldsymbol{Ax} = \boldsymbol{b}$, with $\boldsymbol{A} \in \mathbb{R}^{N \times N}$, $\boldsymbol{x} \in \mathbb{R}^N$, $\boldsymbol{b} \in \mathbb{R}^N$ by minimizing the residual error $||\boldsymbol{b} - \boldsymbol{Ax}||_2$. The idea is to minimize in the kth step of the algorithm the residual $||\boldsymbol{b} - \boldsymbol{Ax}_k||_2$ with $\boldsymbol{x} \in \boldsymbol{x}_0 + K_k(\boldsymbol{A}, \boldsymbol{r}_0) = \boldsymbol{x}_0 + \text{span}\{\boldsymbol{r}_0, \boldsymbol{Ar}_0, ..., \boldsymbol{A}^{k-1}\boldsymbol{r}_0\}$. A space with an architecture like $K_k(\boldsymbol{A}, \boldsymbol{r}_0)$ is called a Krylow subspace. The minimization process can be made efficient by using an orthonormal basis $\{\boldsymbol{v}_1, .., \boldsymbol{v}_k\}$ of the Krylow subspace $K_k(\boldsymbol{A}, \boldsymbol{r}_0)$, which is computed by Arnoldi's method which is an algorithm based on the Gram-Schmidt orthonormalization process [5]. Let $\boldsymbol{V}_k$ denote the matrix which columns are the basis vectors, and $\boldsymbol{V}_{k+1}$ is the basis matrix with one additional orthonormal vector. Hence, $\boldsymbol{x}_k$ can be expressed by a sum of the initial value and a linear combination of the basis vectors with $\boldsymbol{y}$ containing the corresponding coefficients:

$$\boldsymbol{x}_k = \boldsymbol{x}_0 + \boldsymbol{V}_k \boldsymbol{y}. \tag{2.106}$$

There exists a matrix $\boldsymbol{H}_k$, such that $\boldsymbol{AV}_k = \boldsymbol{V}_{k+1}\boldsymbol{H}_k$ and $\boldsymbol{H}_k \in \mathbb{R}^{(k+1)\times N}$ is an upper Hessenberg matrix[3] expanded with an row, which is empty except for the last entry. It can be shown that [64]

$$||\boldsymbol{b} - \boldsymbol{Ax}_k||_2 = ||\,||\boldsymbol{r}_0||_2\,\boldsymbol{e}_1 - \boldsymbol{H}_k\boldsymbol{y}||_2 = J(\boldsymbol{y}), \tag{2.107}$$

where $\boldsymbol{e}_1 = (1, 0, ..., 0)^T \in \mathbb{R}^N$. Hence, the kth iterative solution is $\boldsymbol{x}_k = \boldsymbol{x}_0 + \boldsymbol{V}_k\boldsymbol{y}_k$, where $\boldsymbol{y}_k$ minimizes $J(\boldsymbol{y})$. This minimization process can easily be implemented using a factorization $\boldsymbol{Q}_k\boldsymbol{H}_k = \boldsymbol{R}_k$ achieved with plane rotation, where $\boldsymbol{Q}_k \in \mathbb{R}^{(k+1)\times(k+1)}$ is a rotation matrix and $\boldsymbol{R}_k \in \mathbb{R}^{(k+1)\times k}$ is an upper triangular matrix which last row is zero. Because $\boldsymbol{Q}_k$ is unitary the minimization equation becomes

$$J(\boldsymbol{y}) = ||\,||\boldsymbol{r}_0||_2\,\boldsymbol{e}_1 - \boldsymbol{H}_k\boldsymbol{y}||_2 = ||\boldsymbol{Q}_k[||\boldsymbol{r}_0||_2\,\boldsymbol{e}_1 - \boldsymbol{H}_k\boldsymbol{y}]||_2 = ||\boldsymbol{g}_k - \boldsymbol{R}_k\boldsymbol{y}||_2, \tag{2.108}$$

with $\boldsymbol{g}_k = \boldsymbol{Q}_k\,||\boldsymbol{r}_0||_2\,\boldsymbol{e}_1$. Since the last row of $\boldsymbol{R}_k$ is zero, minimizing $\boldsymbol{y}_k$ is well-defined by $\tilde{\boldsymbol{g}}_k = \tilde{\boldsymbol{R}}_k\boldsymbol{y}_k$ where $\tilde{\boldsymbol{g}}_k$ is the same vector as $\boldsymbol{g}_k$, but the last term is excluded as well as in $\tilde{\boldsymbol{R}}_k$ the last row of $\boldsymbol{R}_k$ is excluded. The residual $||\boldsymbol{g}_k - \boldsymbol{R}_k\boldsymbol{y}_k||_2$ is equal to the absolute value of the last component of $\boldsymbol{g}_k$.
Especially about the GMRES algorithm is that the iterative $\boldsymbol{x}_k$ is not explicitly computed each iteration step, but the coefficient vector $\boldsymbol{y}_k$ and the residual. If the residual becomes small enough, the solution can be computed by a linear combination using $\boldsymbol{y}_k$.
With rising iteration number the computational costs per step increase. To circumvent high computational costs the GMRES algorithm can be stopped after m iterations and restarted with the last iterative solution as initial guess. The restarted algorithm is called GMRES(m). The pseudocode of the GMRES(m) algorithm is given below.

---

[3] An upper Hessenberg matrix is a quadratic matrix, where all entries underneath the first subdiagonal are zero,

e.g. $\begin{pmatrix} \times & \times & \times & \times \\ \times & \times & \times & \times \\ 0 & \times & \times & \times \\ 0 & 0 & \times & \times \end{pmatrix}$

Data: $\boldsymbol{A} \in \mathbb{R}^{N \times N}$, $\boldsymbol{b} \in \mathbb{R}^N$, $\boldsymbol{x}_0 \in \mathbb{R}^N$, tol, restart value m
Result: solution $\boldsymbol{x}$
Initialization: $\boldsymbol{r}_0 = \boldsymbol{b} - \boldsymbol{A}\boldsymbol{x}_0$, $\boldsymbol{v}_1 = \frac{\boldsymbol{r}_0}{||\boldsymbol{r}_0||_2}$, $\gamma_1 = \gamma_{k+1} = ||\boldsymbol{r}_0||_2$;
while $|\gamma_{k+1}| > tol$ **do**
 for $j = 1, ..., m$ **do**
  for $i = 1, ..., j$ **do**
   $h_{ij} = \boldsymbol{v}_i^T \boldsymbol{A}\, \boldsymbol{v}_j$;
  end

  $\hat{\boldsymbol{v}}_{j+1} = \boldsymbol{A}\, \boldsymbol{v}_j - \sum_{i=1}^{j} h_{ij}\boldsymbol{v}_i$;
  $h_{j+1,j} = ||\hat{\boldsymbol{v}}_{j+1}||_2$;
  $\boldsymbol{v}_{j+1} = \frac{1}{h_{j+1,j}}\hat{\boldsymbol{v}}_{j+1}$;
  for $i = 1, ..., j - 1$ **do**
   $\begin{pmatrix} h_{ij} \\ h_{i+1,j} \end{pmatrix} = \begin{pmatrix} c_{i+1} & s_{i+1} \\ -s_{i+1} & c_{i+1} \end{pmatrix} \begin{pmatrix} h_{ij} \\ h_{i+1,j} \end{pmatrix}$;
  end
  $\beta = \sqrt{h_{jj}^2 + h_{j+1,j}^2}$, $s_{j+1} = \frac{h_{j+1,j}}{\beta}$, $c_{j+1} = \frac{h_{jj}}{\beta}$, $h_{jj} = \beta$, $\gamma_{j+1} = -s_{j+1} + \gamma_j$,
  $\gamma_j = c_{j+1}\gamma_j$;
 end
 for $i = j : 1$ **do**
  $y_i = \frac{1}{h_{ii}}\left[\gamma_i - \sum_{k=i+1}^{j} h_{ik}y_k\right]$;
 end

 $\boldsymbol{x} = \boldsymbol{x}_0 + \sum_{i=1}^{j} y_i\, \boldsymbol{v}_i$;
end

Algorithm 2: GMRES(m)

The GMRES linear solver is in general combined with a preconditioner to speed up, which the next chapter deals with.

Preconditioning

A linear system $\boldsymbol{A}\boldsymbol{x} = \boldsymbol{b}$ with $\boldsymbol{A} \in \mathbb{R}^{N \times N}$, $\boldsymbol{x} \in \mathbb{R}^N$, $\boldsymbol{b} \in \mathbb{R}^N$ may become perturbed due to perturbations in the data resulting from uncertainties in the measurements or round off errors

$$\boldsymbol{A}(\boldsymbol{x} + \partial\boldsymbol{x}) = \boldsymbol{A}\boldsymbol{x} + \boldsymbol{A}\partial\boldsymbol{x} = \boldsymbol{b} + \partial\boldsymbol{b}, \tag{2.109}$$

with disturbances $\partial\boldsymbol{x}$ and $\partial\boldsymbol{b}$ in the solution vector or the right hand side respectively. $\boldsymbol{A}\boldsymbol{x} = \boldsymbol{b}$ then yields

$$||\boldsymbol{b}||_2 = ||\boldsymbol{A}\boldsymbol{x}||_2 \leq ||\boldsymbol{A}||_2\, ||\boldsymbol{x}||, \tag{2.110}$$

with the matrix norm defined by

$$||\boldsymbol{A}||_2 = \max_{\boldsymbol{x} \in \mathbb{R}^N, ||\boldsymbol{x}||_2 = 1} ||\boldsymbol{A}\boldsymbol{x}||_2. \tag{2.111}$$

It follows that

$$\frac{1}{||\boldsymbol{x}||_2} \leq \frac{||\boldsymbol{A}||_2}{||\boldsymbol{b}||_2}. \tag{2.112}$$

With $\boldsymbol{A}\partial\boldsymbol{x} = \partial\boldsymbol{b} \Leftrightarrow \partial\boldsymbol{x} = \boldsymbol{A}^{-1}\partial\boldsymbol{b}$, it follows that

$$||\partial\boldsymbol{x}||_2 \leq ||\boldsymbol{A}^{-1}||_2\,||\partial\boldsymbol{b}||_2. \tag{2.113}$$

Combining these two equations yields

$$\frac{||\partial\boldsymbol{x}||_2}{||\boldsymbol{x}||_2} = ||\boldsymbol{A}||_2\,||\boldsymbol{A}^{-1}||_2\,\frac{||\partial\boldsymbol{b}||_2}{||\boldsymbol{b}||_2} = \kappa(\boldsymbol{A})\,\frac{||\partial\boldsymbol{b}||_2}{||\boldsymbol{b}||_2}. \tag{2.114}$$

$\kappa(\boldsymbol{A}) = ||\boldsymbol{A}||_2\,||\boldsymbol{A}^{-1}||_2$ is called *condition number* and is a property of the matrix $\boldsymbol{A}$. As the relation (2.114) shows, the condition number measures the sensitivity of the matrix to errors in the data. A high condition number means that the error of the solution may become high as well. Matrices with a high condition number are called *ill-conditioned*, those with a low condition number *well-conditioned* [14].
A preconditioner $\boldsymbol{P}$ is introduced to the linear system to decrease the condition number of the system matrix $\boldsymbol{A}$ and reduce the error of the solution $\frac{||\partial\boldsymbol{x}||_2}{||\boldsymbol{x}||_2}$ leading to faster convergence behavior. The system matrix can either be preconditioned from the right by solving

$$\boldsymbol{A}\boldsymbol{P}^{-1}\boldsymbol{y} = \boldsymbol{b} \tag{2.115}$$

for $\boldsymbol{y}$ and

$$\boldsymbol{P}\boldsymbol{y} = \boldsymbol{x} \tag{2.116}$$

for $\boldsymbol{x}$ instead of the original system.
Preconditioning from the left results in solving the system

$$\boldsymbol{P}^{-1}(\boldsymbol{A}\boldsymbol{x} - \boldsymbol{b}) = 0. \tag{2.117}$$

Preconditioners can be used to solve a linear system iteratively by applying

$$\boldsymbol{x}_1 = \boldsymbol{x}_0 + \boldsymbol{P}^{-1}(\boldsymbol{b} - \boldsymbol{A}\boldsymbol{x}_0) \tag{2.118}$$

until convergence is reached. The choice of the form of the preconditioner $\boldsymbol{P}$ should be made with respect to

1. The condition number of $\boldsymbol{A}\boldsymbol{P}$, $\boldsymbol{P}^{-1}\boldsymbol{A}$, respectively should be smaller than the one of $\boldsymbol{A}$,

2. The preconditioner should be computational cheap to construct and apply.

Benzi [6] gives a good overview of many different preconditioners. Within this work there are four different preconditioning matrices in usage:

1. The successive over-relaxation (SOR)

$$\boldsymbol{P}_{\text{SOR}} = \boldsymbol{L} + \frac{\boldsymbol{D}}{\omega} \tag{2.119}$$

2. The SORU method

$$\boldsymbol{P}_{\text{SORU}} = \boldsymbol{G} + \frac{\boldsymbol{D}}{\omega} \tag{2.120}$$

3. The symmetric successive over-relaxation (SSOR), which is a SOR sweep combined with a SORU sweep

$$\boldsymbol{P}_{\text{SSOR}} = \frac{\omega}{2 - \omega}(\frac{\boldsymbol{D}}{\omega} - \boldsymbol{L})\boldsymbol{D}^{-1}(\frac{\boldsymbol{D}}{\omega} - \boldsymbol{G}) \tag{2.121}$$

4. The symmetric Gauss-Seidel (SGS), which is a SSOR with $\omega = 1$

$$P_{\mathrm{SGS}} = (D - L)D^{-1}(D - G),$$ (2.122)

where D is a matrix containing the diagonal part of A, L is the lower triangular part of A and G is the upper triangular part and ω is a relaxation parameter. The preconditioning techniques SOR line and symmetric coupled Gauss-Seidel (SCGS) are also used, which means that in the case of SOR Line at first some degrees of freedom are grouped together and SOR or SORU preconditioning is applied to each group separately, details on the grouping based on lines, which connect nodes that are relatively close to another, can be found in [38]. After the separated preconditioning a few steps of SSOR preconditioning are performed. In the SCGS method also a grouping is performed and the SGS preconditioning is applied to every group separately, see [54] for further details.

These preconditioners are used within a preconditioning technique called geometric multigrid. The error of an iterative solution x_k can be defined as $e_k = x - x_k$, where x is the true solution. Briggs [11] shows that an iterative process is effectively in reducing the oscillatory part of the error e, but preserves the smooth parts. The idea of geometric multigrid is to use one of the described preconditioners to reduce the oscillatory part of the error and then coarsen the mesh on which the solution shall be acquired. The coarsened grid has less effort to be computed and can be solved using a direct solver. Geometric multigrid is explained in [11]. The principle is summarized in the following.

Let T_0 denote the fine mesh on which the solution shall be computed and T_1 a coarsened mesh that has half the nodes than the fine one. Solutions have to be mapped from one mesh to another by interpolation, in the case of transforming from a coarser mesh to a finer one this is called prolongation an done by a matrix M for the transformation from T_1 to T_0. In the other way the transformation is called restriction and performed by M^T. The process of multigrid preconditioning can be described by the following pseudocode:

Data: system matrix A_0 on the fine grid and A_1 on the coarse grid, b_0 the right hand side, iterative solution x_0, prolongation matrix M, presmoother, postsmoother, iteration number m_1 and m_2

Result: iterative solution with reduced error x_0

for $i = 1 : m_1$ **do**
   | perform presmoothing;
end
compute residual $r_0 = b_0 - A_0 x_0$;
project residual $r_1 = M^T r_0$;
solve $A_1 x_1 = r_1$ with a direct solver;
map coarse grid correction $x_0 = x_0 + M x_1$;
for $i = 1 : m_2$ **do**
   | perform postsmoothing;
end

Algorithm 3: geometric multigrid preconditioning

2.2.4 Accuracy of CFD

In this section some remarks on the accuracy of CFD as numerical simulation method shall be given. As already outlined in the beginning of this chapter CFD consists of the three main parts:

1. The mathematical model

2. The discretization and

3. The numerical solution.

Hence, there are also three types of errors occurring.

Modeling errors can be defined as the difference between the actual, real flow and the simulated flow resulting from the exact solution of the mathematical model.

Discretization errors are the difference between the exact solution of the mathematical model and the exact solution of the algebraic system resulting from the discretization.

Iteration errors or convergence errors can be defined as difference between the exact solution and the iterative solution of the algebraic system.

To reduce the modeling errors it is necessary to choose appropriate governing equations concerning whether the flow can be treated as laminar or turbulence models have to be used, and whether it is steady or non-stationary, etc. To check the validity of the used model the true flow characteristic has to be known by experimental investigations for example.

In order to evaluate the discretization error it is in good practice to perform a grid convergence study [27]. The simulation is performed on one grid following the grid is refined and a second solution is computed that is compared to the first one. If the difference between both is in an acceptable space the solution concerning the first grid can be used, the solution is said to be *grid independent*.

The last type of error, the convergence error, can be controlled by setting the tolerances for the estimated convergence errors in the iterative solution process.

3 Material and Methods

This chapter is subdivided into three parts. The first part deals with the preprocessing of the image data of an OSAHS patient to gain a suitable model on which fluid flow computations can be performed. The pharyngeal lumen has to be extracted from medical image data and be transferred in a digital representation. The second chapter describes the CFD simulations concerning the used models and boundary conditions. The last part of this chapter describes a comparison study of simulations with an experimental setup as validation basis. Because of missing suitable data of experiments on real pharyngeal anatomies an experiment was chosen which aims at simulating blood flow in an artery with a stenosis. That is a comparable setup to the situation of a constricted pharynx.

3.1 Preprocessing

The base for the digital model of the pharyngeal lumen are two cone beam computed tomography images of the same patient suffering from OSAHS. One image shows the natural anatomical geometry of that patient and the other one was acquired with the patient wearing a mandibular advancement appliance (MAA). A segmentation has been performed of the air lumen in the patient's from the upper hard palate in the nasopharynx to the lower end of the second cervical. The images as well as the segmentation are courtesy of the SICAT GmbH & Co. KG [70]. The images have a size of $512\times512\times512$ voxels, with a voxel extension of $0.3\,\mathrm{mm}$ in each direction. The segmentation was performed in a reduced resolution of $128\times128\times128$ to save computational costs. The segmentation was performed by a watershed algorithm. The idea of this segmentation process is to imagine the grayscale image as a topological surface, where high values correspond to mountains and low values to valleys. The surface is step-by-step filled with water, so that water basins starting from local minima are formed. If two basins would mix together, a separation line is introduced. The different water basins form the segmented areas of the image. Meyer [52] presents some different implementation approaches for the watershed segmentation. A simple pseudocode example is given in the following.

Data: Grayscale image I with value $I(p)$ at voxel p; set of already labeled voxels P
Result: labeled image
for *every voxel $p \in P$* **do**
 | insert all neighbors of p in the priority queue q;
end
sort priority queue q ascending;
while *q is not empty* **do**
 | chose first voxel p in q;
 | **if** *all neighbors that are already labeled have the same label i* **then**
 | | assign label i to voxel p;
 | | insert all not-labeled neighbors of p to the priority queue q;
 | **end**
 | remove voxel p from q;
end

Algorithm 4: Simple example for watershed segmentation

Figure 3.1 shows an overlay of the segmentations of the patient's pharynx with and without MAA. The resolution of the original image is decreased for the overlay propose. On the seg-

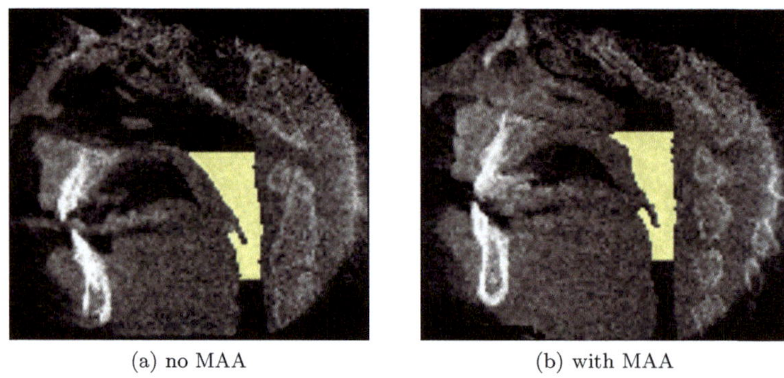

(a) no MAA   (b) with MAA

Figure 3.1: Overlay of segmented pharyngeal lumen and the cone beam computed tomography images with decreased resolution in an sagittal slice.

mented pharynx lumen a surface triangulation is performed to achieve a representation of the surface shape of the patient's pharynx. This is done using MeVisLab, which is a development environment for medical image processing and visualization developed by MeVis Medical Solutions AG and Fraunhofer MEVIS in Bremen, Germany [51]. The surface triangulation was performed by a Marching Cubes Algorithm firstly presented from Lorensen and Cline [17]. The Marching Cubes Algorithm uses cubes, from which each corner is on the cell's midpoint of one voxel. Depending on a threshold for the gray value of the voxel each corner can be grouped in either being inside the element, if the voxel value is smaller, or outside in the other case. There are 8 corners that can have one of these two configurations, which leads to a total number of $2^8 = 256$ different configurations one cube can have. Depending on the configuration triangles are added in the cube separating the inside corners from the outside corners with a normal vector pointing outside the object. These different configurations can effectively be saved in a look-up table LUT. The configuration of each corner inside or outside can be expressed with 0 and 1, which leads to a 8 bit binary number representative for one configuration. The binary number can be used as index for the look-up table, so that LUT(index i) delivers a set of tri-

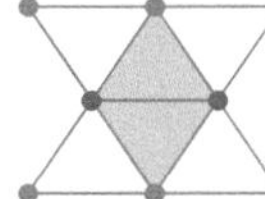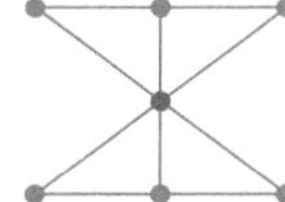

Figure 3.2: The two red vertexes on the left have been contracting resulting in one red vertex on the right with omitting the blue edge and the blue triangles.

angles $t_1, ..., t_m$. Because of rotation symmetry only 15 triangle configurations have to be saved effectively.

The cubes are spread over the image, in that way that each cube has one direct neighbor on every side, meaning both neighboring cubes share 4 corners, or the cube's side is at the boundary of the image. The algorithm is summarized in the following pseudocode:

Data: Grayscale image I with gray value $I(p)$ at voxel p with coordinates x,y,z; a set of neighboring cubes $C = \{c_1, ..., c_n\}$; a threshold τ

Result: set of triangles T

for $i=1{:}n$ **do**

    index=0;

    for $j=1{:}8$ **do**

        Chose corner j of cube i which has the voxel position p_{ij};

        if $I(p_{ij}) < \tau$ **then**

            index$+ = 2^{8-j}$;

        end

    end

    Include all triangles delivered by LUT(index) in the set of triangles T with adjustment of the corner position with respect to the position of cube c_i;

end

Algorithm 5: Marching Cubes Algorithm

The surface triangulation was performed using cubes with a cell extend of one voxel in every spatial direction. The result of the Marching Cubes Algorithm contains many triangles and relies strongly on the cube shape of the voxels. The resulting surface triangulation is very awkward. This awkward shape is not realistic for a smooth human airway tract. The surface triangulation of the pharyngeal lumen is smoothed by reducing the number of triangles, in that kind that two triangle vertices are contracted to one vertex, if they share one edge. The edge and the two belonging triangle faces are removed, see figure 3.2. The contraction is performed until a prescribed percent of triangle reduction is reached. The contracting vertices are chosen with respect to an error based on a quadratic error estimate described by Garland and Heckbert [29]. For a vertex $v = (v_x, v_y, v_z)$ an error is defined based on the planes $ax + by + cz + d = 0$ with $p = [a, b, c, d]^T$, which are the planes of the triangles that intersect the vertex v denoted by planes(v). The error is defined by a squared sum of all intersecting planes

$$\delta(v) = \sum_{p \in \text{planes}(\tilde{v})} (\tilde{v}p)(\tilde{v}p)^T \tag{3.1}$$

$$= \sum_{p \in \text{planes}(\tilde{v})} \tilde{v}pp^T\tilde{v}^T \tag{3.2}$$

$$= \tilde{v}\left(\sum_{p \in \text{planes}(\tilde{v})} K_p\right)\tilde{v}^T \tag{3.3}$$

$$= \tilde{v}Q\tilde{v}^T \tag{3.4}$$

where $\tilde{v} = [v_x, v_y, v_z, 1]^T$ and $K_p = pp^T$. The pseudocode for the triangle reduction is then as follows:

Data: set of triangles with vertices v and planes p, percent of prescribed reduction a

Result: reduced set of triangles

for *every vertex v_i* **do**

    compute matrix $Q_i = \sum\limits_{p \in \text{planes}(v_i)} K_p$;

end

for *any pair (v_1, v_2) that shares an edge* **do**

    compute the optimal contraction target $\bar{v}$ on the edge between v_1 and v_2 by minimizing $\epsilon = \bar{v}(Q_1 + Q_2)\bar{v}^T$;

    set ϵ as the costs for this contraction;

end

sort valid pairs with respect to the costs ϵ beginning with minimal costs;

while $\frac{\text{number of remaining triangles}}{\text{number of initial triangles}} > 1 - a$ **do**

    contract first pair in the sorted list and remove it from list;

    update all costs ϵ involving the contracted vertices;

end

Algorithm 6: Triangle reduction algorithm

The reduction of both surface triangulations is performed with a reduction of $a = 0.75$. The surface triangulation of the pharyngeal lumen without MAA is reduced to a total number of 1854 triangles and 929 vertices and the pharynx with MAA to 3058 triangles and 1531 vertices. After the reduction of the number of the triangles the surface triangulation is additionally smoothed by a Laplacian smoothing which moves a vertex v in direction of the centroid of all vertices it shares edges with. Those are called *adjacent* vertices. Let adj(v) denote the set of adjacent vertices of vertex v. The total number of vertices and triangles is preserved. A relaxation parameter α determines the fraction of the movement in the centroid direction. The smoothing is performed iteratively for m steps. The pseudocode algorithm is as follows.

Data: vertices $\boldsymbol{v}$; number of iterations m; relaxation parameter α
Result: moved vertices $\boldsymbol{v}$
for *i=1:m* **do**
    for *all vertices* $\boldsymbol{v}_i$ **do**
$$\boldsymbol{p} = \frac{1}{|\mathrm{adj}(\boldsymbol{v}_i)|} \sum_{\boldsymbol{v}_j \in \, \mathrm{adj}(\boldsymbol{v}_i)} \boldsymbol{v}_j;$$
$$\boldsymbol{v}_i = \boldsymbol{v}_i + \alpha(\boldsymbol{p} - \boldsymbol{v}_i);$$
    end
end

Algorithm 7: Laplacian surface triangulation smoothing

The Laplacian smoothing was preformed with an iteration number of $m = 5$ and a relaxation parameter of $\alpha = 0.2$. Figure 3.3 shows results of the different steps from the segmentation to the preprocessed surface triangulation for both datasets.

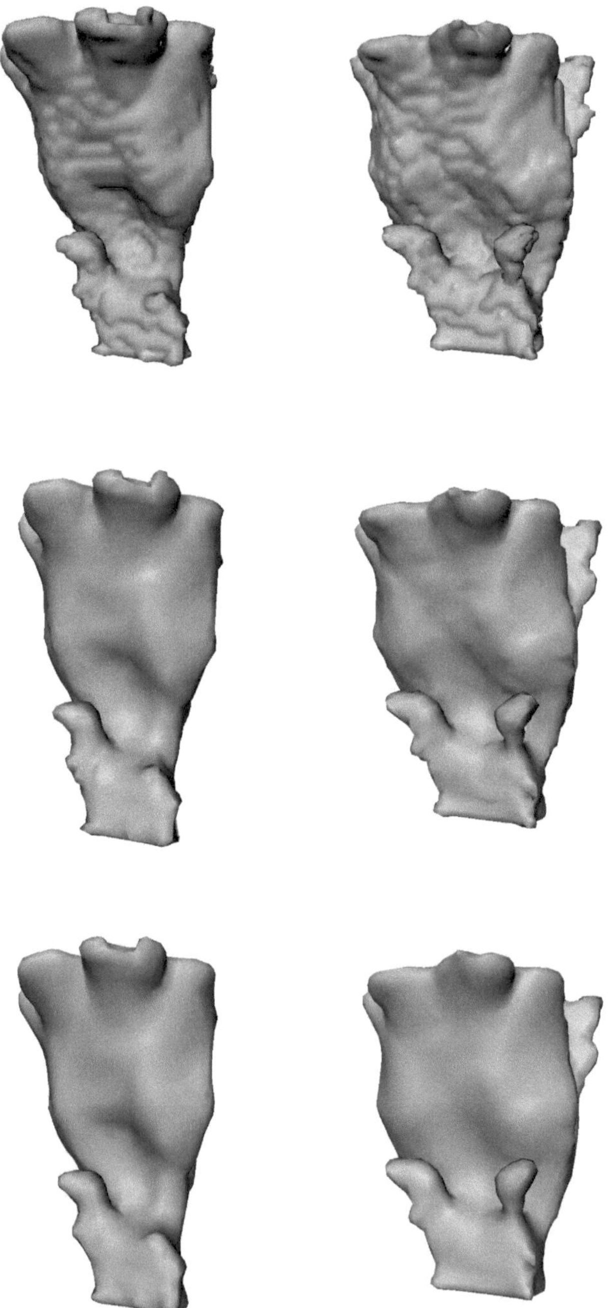

Figure 3.3: On the left hand side the surface triangulation of the patient's pharyngeal lumen without MAA is shown and on the right with MAA. The triangulations in the first row are the results from the Marching Cubes Algorithm with cubes of one voxel cell extend in each spatial direction. In the second row the triangulations are shown after a reduction of triangles by 75%. In the third row the triangulations are visualized after the Laplacian smoothing with an iteration number of 5 and a relaxation parameter of 0.2.

3.2 Simulation

The simulation of airflow in the human pharynx based on an OSAHS patient's data are performed with the COMSOL© software. The preprocessed surface triangulations are therefore imported in COMSOL©, in the following they are called pharynx models. The modeling of the CFD simulation in the human pharynx is explained in the following. At first the physical parameters influencing the flow are described.

Three different types of mathematical models are used to simulate the airflow:

1. The flow is simulated using the Navier Stokes Equations without turbulence modeling (2.26). Within the COMSOL© environment this is denoted with *laminar* solution, although the exact equations that describe the laminar and the turbulent flow are in both cases the same Navier Stokes Equations. Simulating turbulent flow using Navier Stokes Equations without turbulence modeling is limited because of the very high spatial resolution that is required. Therefore that type is denoted with *laminar* in COMSOL©.

2. The flow is simulated using the Reynolds Averaged Navier Stokes Equations and the $k - \epsilon$ turbulence model.

3. The flow is simulated using the Reynolds Averaged Navier Stokes Equations and the $k - \omega$ turbulence model.

Although the Mach numbers are expected to be well below 0.3, the influence of the compressibility of the air was not omitted, which should give more precise results. In all cases the stationary equations are used, because the boundary conditions are static.

The pharynx models are assumed to be comprised of air, which defines the values for the density of the material ρ and the dynamic viscosity μ. The material parameters are defined by build-in functions in COMSOL©, which is for the density of air an analytical function

$$\rho(T/\mathrm{K}, pA/\mathrm{Pa}) = \rho(\tilde{T}, \tilde{pA}) = \frac{\tilde{pA}}{\tilde{T}} \cdot \frac{0.02897}{8.314} \cdot \mathrm{kg\,m}^3 \qquad (3.5)$$

dependent on the temperature T and the pressure pA, and a piece-wise function for the dynamic viscosity

$$\mu(T/\mathrm{K}) = \mu(\tilde{T}) = -\,8.38278 \cdot 10^{-7} + 8.35717342 \cdot 10^{-8}\,\tilde{T} - 7.69429583 \cdot 10^{-11}\,\tilde{T}^2 \qquad (3.6)$$
$$+\ 4.6437266 \cdot 10^{-14}\,\tilde{T}^3 - 1.06585607 \cdot 10^{-17}\,\tilde{T}^4 \cdot \mathrm{Pa} \cdot \mathrm{s}$$

dependent on the temperature T. The pressure was set to atmospheric pressure $pA = 1\,\mathrm{atm} = 1.0133 \cdot 10^5\,\mathrm{Pa}$ and the temperature was set to $T = 34°\,\mathrm{C} = 307.15\,\mathrm{K}$, which Keck et al. [40] measured as mean temperature value in the nasopharynx in 50 volunteers. This leads to the parameters $\rho = 1.1495\,\mathrm{kg\,m}^3$ and $\mu = 1.8823 \cdot 10^{-5}\,\mathrm{Pa} \cdot \mathrm{s}$.

In the case of stationary, compressible, viscous flow the governing equations have got elliptic character. Therefore boundary conditions have to be prescribed on the whole closed boundary: The surface of the pharyngeal air volume $\partial\Omega$ is divided in three different types of boundary conditions: an inlet area Γ_{in}, an outlet area Γ_{out} and a no-slip wall Γ_{wall}, with $\Gamma_{\mathrm{in}} \cup \Gamma_{\mathrm{out}} \cup \Gamma_{\mathrm{wall}} = \partial\Omega$ and $\Gamma_{\mathrm{in}} \cap \Gamma_{\mathrm{out}} = \emptyset$, $\Gamma_{\mathrm{in}} \cap \Gamma_{\mathrm{wall}} = \emptyset$, $\Gamma_{\mathrm{out}} \cap \Gamma_{\mathrm{wall}} = \emptyset$. The no-slip wall means that the fluid at the solid wall is not moving leading to the Dirichlet's boundary condition

$$\boldsymbol{u}(x, y, z) = \boldsymbol{0}\ \mathrm{ms}^{-1}\ \text{for}\ (x, y, z) \in \Gamma_{\mathrm{wall}}. \qquad (3.7)$$

For the inlet and outlet boundary conditions two different combinations were tested:

1. A volume flow rate is prescribed at the inlet and zero pressure at the outlet, as Fan et al. [26] used it for their simulation. They used a flow rate of $300\,\mathrm{mls}^{-1}$. Shome et al. [69] reported a mean flow rate at the inlet of the pharynx of $400\,\mathrm{mls}^{-1}$, which was used in the simulation within this work as well. The velocity at the inlet was prescribed using the volume flow rate. The velocity is prescribed to be $u_{in} = \phi\,A^{-1}$ in axial direction of the pharynx, which is the $-z$ direction, where ϕ is the prescribed inlet volume rate and A the inlet area. The velocity in the other directions is zero at the inlet. The complete set of Dirichlet's boundary conditions in the first case are

$$\boldsymbol{u}(x,y,z) = \mathbf{0}\ \mathrm{ms}^{-1} \text{ for } (x,y,z) \in \Gamma_{\mathrm{wall}} \tag{3.8}$$

$$\boldsymbol{u}(x,y,z) = \begin{pmatrix} 0\,\mathrm{ms}^{-1} \\ 0\,\mathrm{ms}^{-1} \\ -u_{in} \end{pmatrix} \text{ for } (x,y,z) \in \Gamma_{\mathrm{in}}$$

$$p(x,y,z) = 0\,\mathrm{Pa} \text{ for } (x,y,z) \in \Gamma_{\mathrm{out}},$$

which are called boundary type one in the following.

2. In the second case a pressure drop from the inlet to the outlet of the flow is prescribed, which is comparable to the physiological phenomena of the lung establishing a negative pressure during the inhalation process. The same pressure values that used Holsbeke et al. [73] in the flow simulation were prescribed for inlet and outlet boundary conditions for this study as well. This leads to the set of Dirichlet's boundary conditions

$$\boldsymbol{u}(x,y,z) = \mathbf{0}\ \mathrm{ms}^{-1} \text{ for } (x,y,z) \in \Gamma_{\mathrm{wall}} \tag{3.9}$$

$$p(x,y,z) = 0\,\mathrm{Pa} \text{ for } (x,y,z) \in \Gamma_{\mathrm{in}}$$

$$p(x,y,z) = -20\,\mathrm{Pa} \text{ for } (x,y,z) \in \Gamma_{\mathrm{in}},$$

which are called boundary type two in the following.

If a turbulence model is used, turbulence boundary conditions have to be prescribed at the inlet of the flow as well. In the case of unknown turbulence parameters, they can be estimated. The turbulent kinetic energy can be estimated by using the turbulence intensity, which is defined by

$$I = \frac{\bar{u}'}{|\boldsymbol{U}|} = \frac{\sqrt{\frac{1}{3}{u'_x}^2 + {u'_y}^2 + {u'_z}^2}}{|\boldsymbol{U}|} = \frac{\sqrt{\frac{2}{3}k}}{|\boldsymbol{U}|}, \tag{3.10}$$

where $|\boldsymbol{U}|$ is the mean velocity and u'_x, u'_y and u'_z are the turbulent fluctuations. This yields for the turbulent kinetic energy

$$k = \frac{3}{2}(|\boldsymbol{U}|\,I)^2. \tag{3.11}$$

The mean velocity is set to the value u_{in} for both boundary types. The turbulence intensity in the case of prescribed velocity was taken as the same that Holsbeke et al. [73] used, which was $5\,\%$. In the case of prescribed velocity an estimation of the turbulence intensity in a pipe was used [49]

$$I = 0.16\,\mathrm{Re}^{-\frac{1}{8}}, \tag{3.12}$$

the Reynolds number was computed by the hydraulic diameter $L_{in} = 4\,C_{in}\,A_{in}^{-1}$, derived from the inlet area A_{in} and the inlet contour C_{in}, and the prescribed inlet velocity u_{in}.

According to Taylor [72] the dissipation is proportional to the relation of kinetic energy and a turbulence length scale L_T, which is characteristic for the larger eddies:

$$\epsilon \propto \frac{k^{\frac{3}{2}}}{L_T}, \tag{3.13}$$

within this context the inlet dissipation is estimated by

$$\epsilon = C_\mu \frac{k^{\frac{3}{2}}}{L_T}, \tag{3.14}$$

where C_μ is a constant defined in (2.67) and L_T is chosen based on an estimation for pipe flow [49]

$$L_T = 0.07 L_{in}. \tag{3.15}$$

Kolmogorov [43] described the specific dissipation by

$$\omega = c \frac{k^{\frac{1}{2}}}{L_T}, \tag{3.16}$$

where c is a constant. Within this context the inlet specific dissipation was computed by

$$\omega = \frac{k^{\frac{1}{2}}}{(\beta_0^*)^{\frac{1}{4}} L_T}. \tag{3.17}$$

The spatial discretization was performed using the finite element method with linear Lagrangian elements for all dependent variables. Although higher degree polynomials are expected to have a better accuracy, linear polynomials are chosen because higher polynomials introduce more degrees of freedom and CFD simulations need a high spatial resolution, which already lead to a high number of degrees of freedom. Hence, the interpolation functions of the finite element method are chosen to be less computational expensive to enable a higher spatial resolution. Wilcox [76] as well as Ferziger and Perić [27] underline that it is necessary to perform a grid independency study, to evaluate the numerical accuracy of the simulated flow. Although this is an important part of CFD it is sparsely described by many authors. Fan et al. [26] just mentioned that *"mesh independent test was taken"* without giving information on how it was performed. Martonen et al. [50] mentioned that *"large scales of the flow field (i.e., the maximum velocities) and flow patterns were insensitive"*, but not what they defined as insensitive and how the flow might be influenced by the smaller scale dependency. Van Holsbeke et al. [73] said that *"A sensitivity study showed that a computational grid between 500,000 and 1,000,000 tetrahedral cells is sufficient for reaching mesh convergence"*. Vos et al. [74] do not mention a grid sensitivity study at all.

Within this work the dependency of the solutions on the computational grid is evaluated as follows: At first a solution for the velocity u_{coarse} without turbulence model is performed on the model of the pharynx without MAA with the first type of boundary conditions at a coarse grid, which has in total 21,581 quadrahedral and tetrahedral elements. This grid is refined globally one time so it has 57,658 quadrahedral and tetrahedral elements and a solution for the velocity u_{refined} is obtained using the same conditions as for the first one. Two solutions can be compared with respect to a scalar quantity ψ by

$$eps(\psi_0, \psi_1) = \frac{|\psi_0 - \psi_1|}{\max\left(|\psi_0|, |\psi_1|, \delta\right)}, \tag{3.18}$$

where δ is a constant, which should prevent division by zero and the enhancement of errors for small values of ψ. The parameter is chosen to be $\delta = 10^{-4}$. For the two mentioned meshes the velocity magnitude is compared, so $\phi_0 = |\boldsymbol{u}_{\mathrm{coarse}}|$ and $\phi_1 = |\boldsymbol{u}_{\mathrm{refined}}|$. Values within the elements can be interpolated using the finite element node values and the shape functions. This first simulations are performed to identify the area, where the error between the simulations are the highest. This is adapted in the process of mesh generation by forcing the mesh to be more dense there. In the following the strategy is to use a grid that is finer with respect to the initial simulations called mesh M_0 and then this grid is refined one time to mesh M_1 and is then again compared to the coarser solution by (3.18) to estimate the positions and the amount of the highest errors. For the boundary type two meshes with less elements than for the first boundary type were used because of a longer computational time of the simulations with the second boundary type. All meshes are composed of quadrahedral and tetrahedral elements, the sizes of each are summarized in table 3.1.

Table 3.1: Number of mesh elements for the different simulations.

data	boundary type	mesh	number of elements
no MAA	one	M_0	231,207
		M_1	534,589
	two	M_0	198,882
		M_1	231,207
with MAA	one	M_0	373,803
		M_1	587,375
	two	M_0	238,440
		M_1	373,803

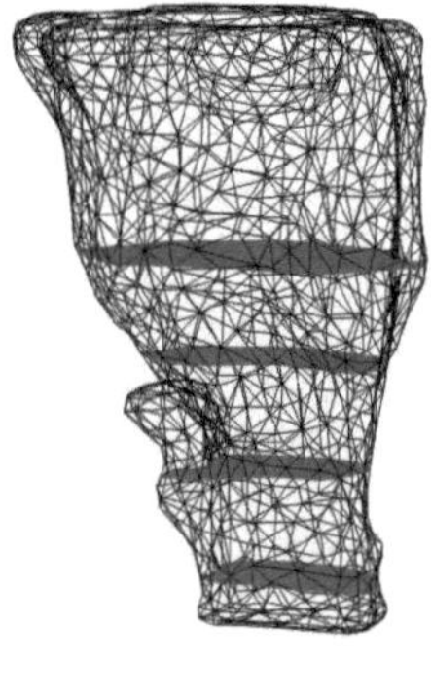

(a) no MAA

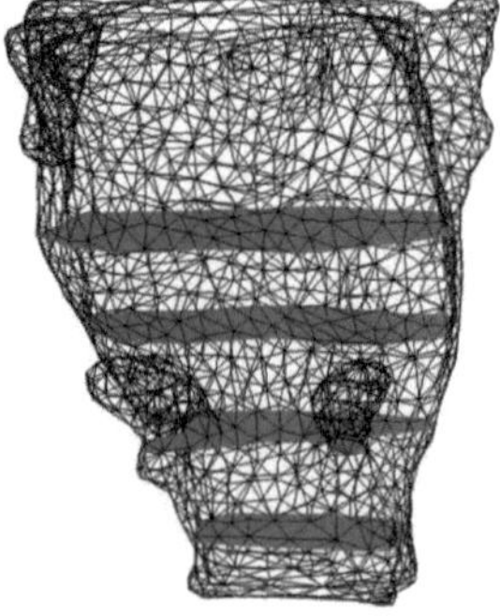

(b) with MAA

Figure 3.4: Visualization of the slices orthogonal to the pharynx axis that are used for the comparison. It should be remarked that no image registration has been performed with the different patient's datasets and there is no direct match between the slices of the two models. Nevertheless they have been chosen in that way that they should represent comparable areas of the two different models.

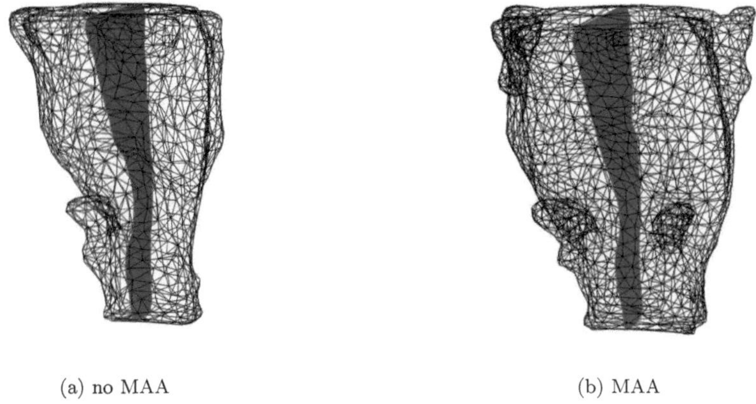

(a) no MAA   (b) MAA

Figure 3.5: Visualization of the axial slice that is used for the comparison. As in the case of the orthogonal slices a direct match between the two axial slices is not given.

Four slices are chosen in each pharyngeal model orthogonal to the pharynx axis, see figure 3.4. The solutions are compared to each other by computing the Reynolds number based on the average velocity of each slice and the average kinematic viscosity and the hydraulic diameter based on the area and the contour of each slice. In each slice also the average pressure was compared. On one slice in the axial direction at the middle of each model, see figure 3.5, the velocity magnitude and the pressure have also been compared. The error estimate (3.18) is used with $\delta = 10^{-4}$ for the comparisons.

For the numerical solution of the simulations with the stationary Navier Stokes Equations the nonlinear damped Newton method was applied. The linearized system of equations has been solved with the iterative GMRES solver, which has been preconditioned with the multigrid technique, where SCGS is used as pre- and as postsmoother, the coarse solution of the multigrid technique is computed with the direct PARDISO solver.

The initial guess is either the zero solution

$$\boldsymbol{u}_0(x, y, z) = 0 \,\mathrm{ms}^{-1}, \; p_0(x, y, z) = 0 \,\mathrm{Pa}, \; (x, y, z) \in \Omega/\partial\Omega \tag{3.19}$$

or if the solution has already been obtained on a coarser grid that one is used as initial guess. A segregated solution process is used to solve the turbulence models which means that two groups are build, one with the velocity and the pressure as dependent variables, and the other one with the turbulent kinetic energy k and the dissipation ϵ respectively the specific dissipation ω. One iteration of solving for the velocity and the pressure is performed with fixed values for k and ϵ resp. ω and afterwards three iterations of solving for k and ϵ resp. ω are performed with fixed values for the velocity and the pressure. This cycle is called one iteration of the segregated solution process. One of the inner iterations contains the solution of the discretized equations with one iteration of the damped Newton method with a constant damping factor of $\lambda = 0.5$, with the iterative GMRES solver and multigrid preconditioning with the PARDISO direct solver for the coarse solution and SCGS pre- and postsmoother for the solution of the velocity and the pressure and three damped Newton iterations with the constant damping factor $\lambda = 0.35$ and SOR line as pre- and postsmoother for the solution of k and ϵ resp. ω. The values for the parameters are summarized in table 3.2. Presented settings are default settings defined by

Table 3.2: parameter values for the numerical solution

parameter	description	value
$\lambda_{\min}$	recovery damping factor for Newton method	0.75
$\lambda_{\min}$	minimal damping factor for Newton method	10^{-6}
itmax	maximal number of Newton iterations	25
tol, tol_1, tol_2	relative tolerances for the Newton method and the GMRES solver	0.001
m	restart GMRES after m iterations	50

COMSOL©.

Kuzmin and Mierka [44] describe that initial conditions of the turbulence parameters can be estimated by

$$k_0 = \left(\frac{\mu}{\rho l_{\mathrm{mix}}}\right)^2 \text{ and } \epsilon_0 = \frac{C_\mu k_0^{\frac{3}{2}}}{l_{\mathrm{mix}}}, \tag{3.20}$$

where l_{mix} is the mixing length. For the initial guesses of the turbulence parameters the implementation provided by COMSOL© assigns a factor to the turbulence kinetic energy, which is then given by

$$k_0 = \left(\frac{10\mu}{\rho l_{\mathrm{mix}}}\right)^2. \tag{3.21}$$

The mixing length is estimated as $0.1\,l_+$, where l_+ is the mixing length limit. The mixing length limit is estimated as the shortest side of the geometry bounding box. The initial guess for the specific dissipation is given by

$$\omega = \frac{k_0^{\frac{1}{2}}}{0.1\,l_+}.\tag{3.22}$$

Some numerical tests are performed with the parameters describing the turbulence statistics at the inlet. Simulations are done with the pharyngeal model without MAA with the turbulence intensity varied by 20 % up and down from the calculated value in the case of prescribed inlet velocity, as well as simulations with the length scale varied by 20 % up and down. In the case of the prescribed inlet pressure the reference velocity for the computation of the kinetic energy, which is set to be u_{in}, is also varied by 20 % up and down. One simulation is performed with boundary type one and 20% increased turbulence intensity on the model with MAA to validate the transferability of the results on the different geometry.

3.3 Experimental Validation

Ferziger and Perić [27] underline the importance of the comparison of fluid flow simulations with experimental data to guarantee the correctness of the simulation. In the case of the human pharynx of a specific patient no such experimental data exists. In the cases were experiments had been performed on modeled human airways ([48], [34]) the description of the used geometry are not as detailed enough to rebuild it accurately to reconstruct the simulations. Nevertheless a comparison of the results of the COMSOL© simulation framework with an experimental data is used to validate accuracy. An experiment of Ahmed and Giddens [2] is chosen to be reconstructed. They examined the behavior of blood flowing through an artery with a stenosis. The case of an arterial stenosis is comparable to the case of the OSAHS disease. Both are characterized by nearly circular shaped pipes, the artery or the pharynx respectively, that exhibit a constriction evoked either by sediments of the blood or the tung.

Ahmed and Giddens constructed circular pipes with different degrees of constriction and examined a water glycerol mixture traveling through this pipe by different Reynolds numbers. The constrictions were build to decrease the pipe's volume in the constriction area by 25%, 50% or 75%. For the numerical simulation the case of a 75% stenosis is chosen. In that case the pipe has a unconstricted diameter of $d = 2\,\text{inch}$ and in the constricted part 1 inch, the area of constriction was 4 inch long. In the experiment the pipe had an axial length of 72 inch after the constriction. In the simulation a pipe of 22 inch axial length was chosen, because the fluid behavior in the very vicinity of the constriction is of interest and the computational costs should be kept as small as possible. The geometry is shown in figure 3.6.

The simulations are performed at a Reynolds number based on the unconstricted pipe diam-

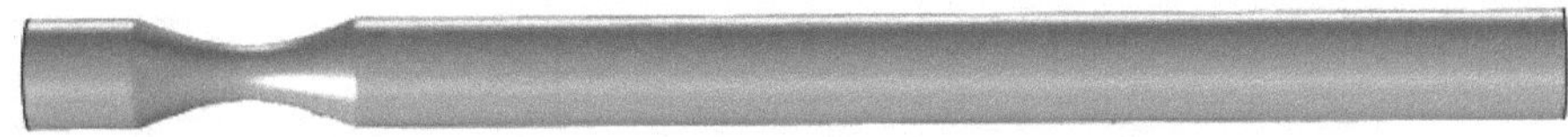

Figure 3.6: Geometry of the reconstructed experimental setup of a 75% arterial stenosis.

eter and the kinematic viscosity $\nu = 0.12 \cdot 10^{-4}\,\mathrm{m^2 s^{-1}}$ of 2000 resulting in an inlet velocity of $u_{\mathrm{in}} = 0.47\,\mathrm{ms^{-1}}$. As no information on the pressure drop were given in the experiment of Ahmed and Giddens the boundary conditions were chosen to resample the first type of boundary conditions that were used to model the fluid flow in the human pharynx. The set of boundary conditions are given by

$$\boldsymbol{u}(x,y,z) = \boldsymbol{0}\ \mathrm{ms}^{-1} \text{ for } (x,y,z) \in \Gamma_{\mathrm{wall}} \tag{3.23}$$

$$\boldsymbol{u}(x,y,z) = \begin{pmatrix} 0\,\mathrm{ms}^{-1} \\ 0\,\mathrm{ms}^{-1} \\ u_{\mathrm{in}} \end{pmatrix} \text{ for } (x,y,z) \in \Gamma_{\mathrm{in}}$$

$$p(x,y,z) = 0\,\mathrm{Pa} \text{ for } (x,y,z) \in \Gamma_{\mathrm{out}}$$

with the pipe's axis pointing in the z-direction.
Ahmed and Giddens mentioned oscillations of the flow further downstream of the constricted area. To capture this behavior a time dependent simulation was performed, no turbulence model was applied, the governing equations are given by (2.24), which are of parabolic type, that have a downstream information distribution. Additionally to the inlet, outlet and slip wall boundary conditions an initial solution has to be prescribed for the first time point. Three simulations on three different meshes are performed, where the first one has the zero solution as initial solution. The two following ones each with refined grid the solution of the last time step of the simulation on the coarser mesh is used as initial flow situation. The mesh sizes are 260,675 elements, 697,212 elements and 857,360 elements. The solution is simulated at time points t in the range from $t_0 = 0\,\mathrm{s}$ to $t_{max} = 5\,\mathrm{s}$ with a step size of $0.2\,\mathrm{s}$. Linear Lagrangian elements are used in the finite element method for the velocity and the pressure. The solution was obtained using the variable step size, variable order backward differentiation algorithm IDA and the GMRES iterative solver with multigrid preconditioning and SCGS as pre- and postsmoother and PARDISO as direct solver for the coarse grid. The parameters are chosen according to table 3.2.
Ahmed and Giddens published the axial velocity component u_z divided by the mean axial inlet velocity $\bar{u}$ at the axial centerline as well as the flow profile of the axial velocity component u_z divided by the mean axial inlet velocity at orthogonal slices with a distance to the constriction of $\Delta z = 0\,\mathrm{m}$, d, $2.5\,d$, $4\,d$, $5\,d$ and $6\,d$. These results are used to compare the numerical simulations with the experimental data.

4 Results

This chapter presents the simulation results obtained for the two different pharyngeal geometries and for the digital replica of the experimental setup of the arterial stenosis. The first section of this chapter deals with the comparison of the simulation with the experimental setup of the stenosis. In the second section the simulations of the airflow in the patient's pharynx are presented. That section is subdivided into two parts: The first part deals with examinations of the solution's grid dependency as well as the influence of the variation of the inlet turbulence statistic parameters: the turbulence intensity, the length scale and the velocity scale. In the second part the difference of fluid flow in the two patient's pharyngeal geometries with and without MAA are compared to each other.

4.1 Comparison to Measurement

The simulation of the fluid flow on the coarsest grid with 260,675 mesh elements in total is depicted in figure 4.1. The velocity in axial direction u_z at the time steps $t \in \{0\,\text{s}, 1\,\text{s}, 2\,\text{s}, 3\,\text{s}, 4\,\text{s}, 5\,\text{s}\}$ is shown. The simulation results of all used time steps can be found in the appendix 7.17 and 7.18.

It shows up that the velocity is the highest in the area of the constriction. The flow appears to reach a stationary state with an asymmetric flow profile. The described transition in the turbulent oscillatory flow by Ahmed and Giddens is not observed in this simulation. The simulation is repeated on a refined mesh with 697,212 mesh elements in total by using the last time step of the simulation on the coarser grid as initial solution. The flow in axial direction is depicted in figure 4.2 at the time points from 0 s to 5 s in 1 s steps. The flow simulations at all time points can be found in the appendix 7.19 and 7.20.

The simulation shows a transition to oscillation, especially in the last time step the flow has an oscillatory profile. With that last time step as initial solution another simulation is performed on a further refined grid. The results are shown in figure 4.3 at the same time points, all time points are depicted in the appendix 7.21 and 7.22.

The simulation shows the described oscillatory flow behavior. The flow velocity is the highest in the area of the constriction and decreases the most at the beginning of the oscillation, as it was described in the experimental study [2]. In this case the turbulent behavior could be simulated quite well using the Navier Stokes Equations without turbulence modeling, which shows that those simulations are not restricted to laminar flow as the denomination in the COMSOL© software environment could lead to believe.

The simulation results on the finest grid are used for the comparison to the experimental data concerning the flow velocity profile orthogonal to the axial direction. Ahmed and Giddens published the time averaged axial velocity at different distances $\Delta z \in \{0\,\text{m}, d, 2.5\,d, 4\,d, 5\,d, 6\,d\}$ to the constriction. The time average of the simulation is performed using the last time steps from $t = 4\,\text{s}$ to $t = 5\,\text{s}$ in 0.2 s steps, which are depicted in figure 4.4, the positions of the examined slices are denoted with white lines. The time average is restricted to the last simulated second to reduce the influence of flow velocities that are produced in a not fully developed transitional state. The comparison is depicted in figure 4.5.

The simulation and the experimental data show a close match in most cases, only the simulated velocity of the slice at distance $\Delta z = 2.5\,d$ is not as high as in the experimental setup. The flow velocity at the slice with distance $\Delta z = d$ in the center of the pipe is lower than in the experiments. This results from the slight asymmetry of the simulated flow profile that still appears in the finest spatial discretization.

The comparison of the arterial stenosis replica and the pharyngeal geometries it shows up that the extend of the computational area of the pharyngeal geometries after the most constricted part is smaller than the extend of the computational domain of the arterial stenosis. Therefore the results of the the first two slices showing in the most a good match are more meaningful for this application. It appears that the flow before, in and directly after the constriction is stationary, which makes the use of stationary simulations in the pharyngeal geometries justifiable.

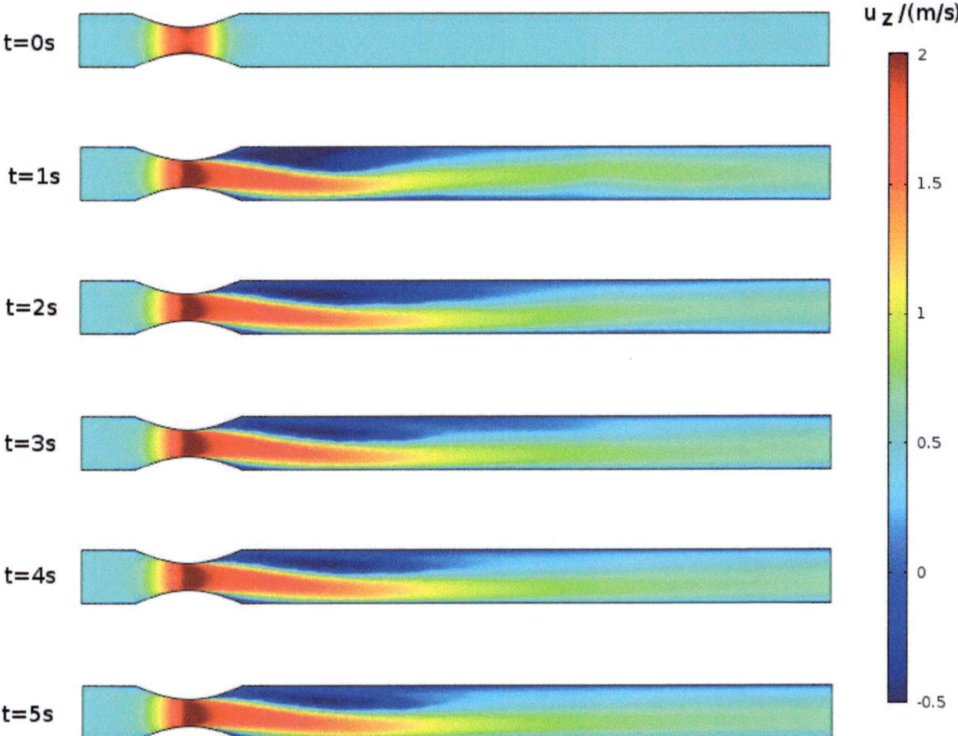

Figure 4.1: Simulation results for the stenosis model for the grid with 260,675 mesh elements for the time points $t \in \{0\,\mathrm{s}, 1\,\mathrm{s}, 2\,\mathrm{s}, 3\,\mathrm{s}, 4\,\mathrm{s}, 5\,\mathrm{s}\}$.

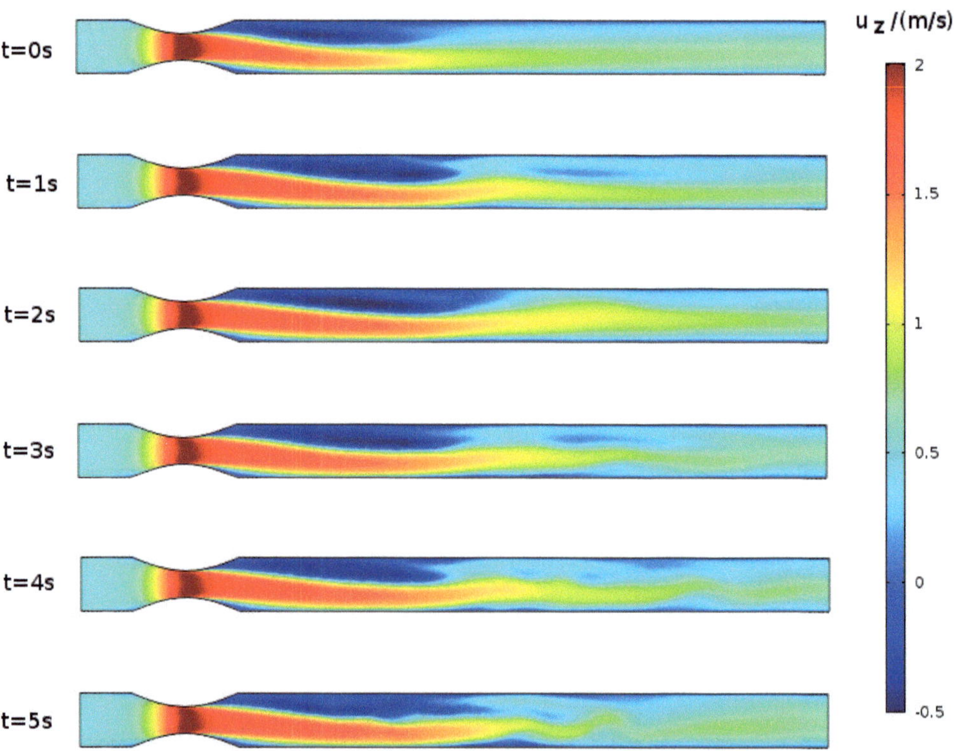

Figure 4.2: Simulation results for the stenosis model for the grid with 697,212 mesh elements for the time points $t \in \{0\,\mathrm{s}, 1\,\mathrm{s}, 2\,\mathrm{s}, 3\,\mathrm{s}, 4\,\mathrm{s}, 5\,\mathrm{s}\}$.

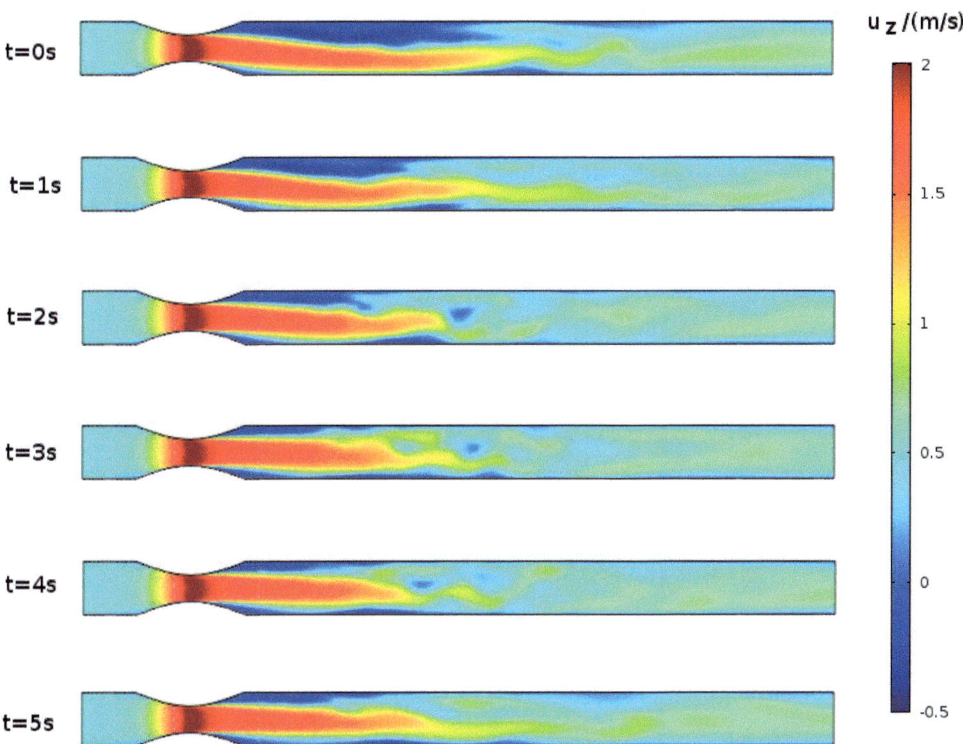

Figure 4.3: Simulation results for the stenosis model for the grid with 857,360 mesh elements for the time points $t \in \{0\,\mathrm{s}, 1\,\mathrm{s}, 2\,\mathrm{s}, 3\,\mathrm{s}, 4\,\mathrm{s}, 5\,\mathrm{s}\}$.

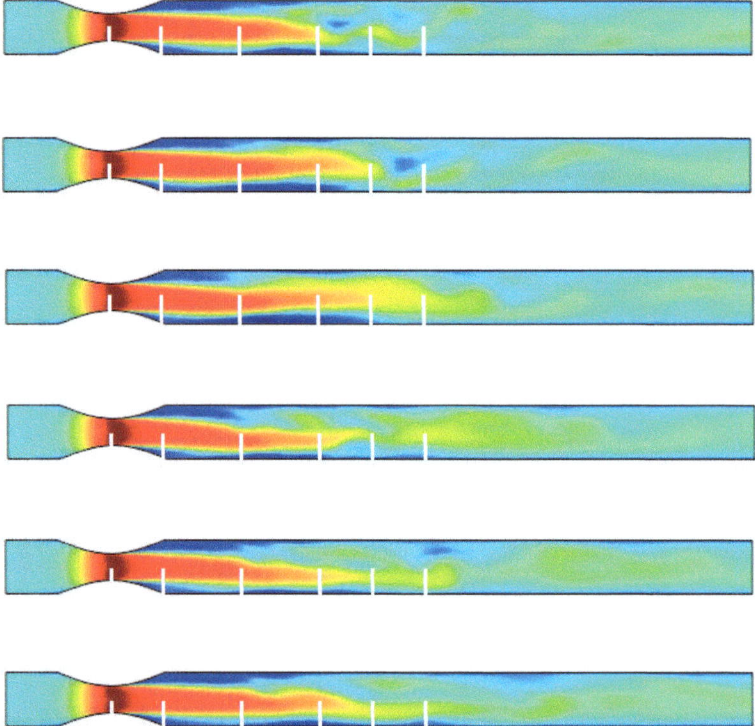

Figure 4.4: Simulation results for the stenosis model for the grid with 857,360 mesh elements for the time points $t \in \{4\,\text{s}, 4.2\,\text{s}, 4.4\,\text{s}, 4.6\,\text{s}, 4.8\,\text{s}, 5\,\text{s}\}$. The orthogonal slices that are used for the comparison of the velocity profiles are marked with white lines.

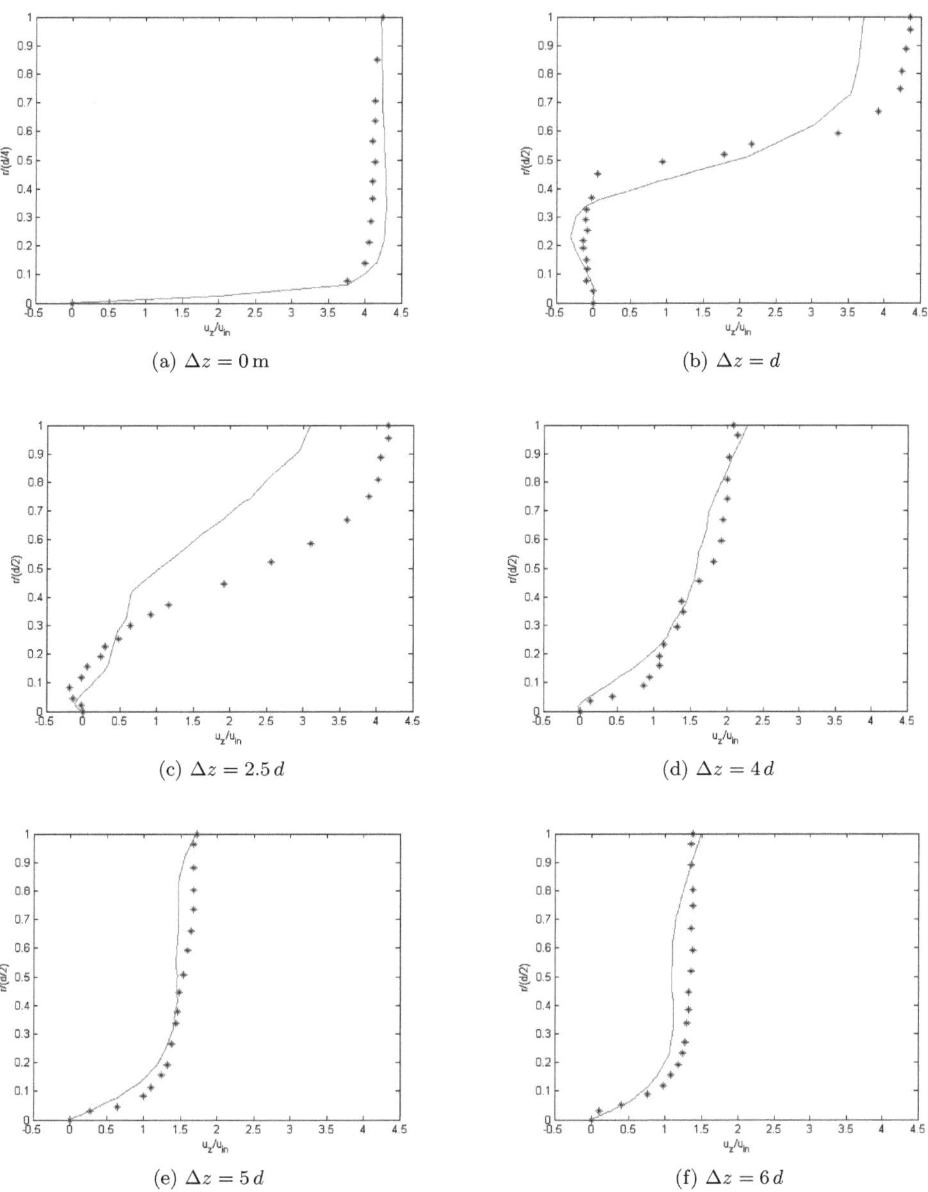

(a) $\Delta z = 0\,\mathrm{m}$

(b) $\Delta z = d$

(c) $\Delta z = 2.5\,d$

(d) $\Delta z = 4\,d$

(e) $\Delta z = 5\,d$

(f) $\Delta z = 6\,d$

Figure 4.5: Comparison of the measurement data marked with blue stars with the simulation results visualized with a red line of the flow profile in different distances Δz to the most constricted part. The flow velocity divided by the prescribed inlet velocity is depicted on the x-axis and the distance to the wall r divided by the radius of the pipe is on the y-axis. It should be noted that the radius in the constriction plane is only half times the pipe's radius.

4.2 Pharyngeal Flow Simulation

Simulations in the pharynx of two different patient data sets of the same patient one with and the other without a MAA are preformed with two different types of boundary conditions. In this section the dependency of the simulation results on the used grid size is evaluated in the first part. This evaluation is used in the comparison of the flow in the two different geometries in the second part of this chapter.

4.2.1 Grid Dependency

Simulations are performed on a coarse grid and a globally refined grid and the velocity magnitude is compared for both simulations with respect to the error measure *eps* (3.18) to identify areas with the highest differences. The results are depicted in figure 4.6. It shows up that the error is the highest in and under the constriction. The meshes are adapted to that behavior in that kind that they are relatively coarse above the stenotic area and fine in and underneath the most constricted part. The meshes that are used for the different simulations are depicted in figure 4.7 for the pharyngeal geometry without MAA and in figure 4.8 with MAA.

A solution in which all dependent variables - the three velocity components, the pressure, the kinetic energy k per unit mass and the dissipation ϵ or the specific dissipation rate ω respectively - do not vary in the whole domain, was not reachable with the used geometries. Therefore the error with respect to the error measure *eps* (3.18) has been computed for the variables and positions that are used for the comparison of the two different pharyngeal geometries in the second part of this chapter. The idea is to identify with the grid dependency study parameters, that are reliable, because they do not change much in simulations with different mesh sizes, and use that parameters for the evaluation of the flow in geometries with and without MAA.

Simulations are performed with the two different geometries, two different boundary condition types and three different types of mathematical models: the Navier Stokes Equations, the Reynolds Averaged Navier Stokes Equations with $k - \epsilon$ turbulence model and $k - \omega$ turbulence model. But for both pharyngeal geometries no solution could be obtained without using a turbulence model in the case of boundary type two, the prescribed pressure drop. The computation failed because convergence could not be reached within the maximal number of iterations of the nonlinear Newton solver.

The behavior in grid dependency is quite the same for the two turbulence models and the Navier Stokes Equations in the case of boundary condition type one. Therefore only the results obtained with the $k - \omega$ model are presented in this section and used for the comparison. The results of both other mathematical models can be found in the appendix in figure 7.1 to figure 7.3.

In figure 4.9 the differences with respect to the error measure *eps* (3.18) are depicted for the velocity magnitude in the axial slice as well as the pressure in the axial slice and on the surface of the pharyngeal geometry without MAA. It should be noted that the error is visualized within the boundaries of 0 to 1 for the velocity magnitude and from 0 to 2 for the pressure, because whereas the velocity magnitude can only have positive values the pressure can be negative as well and therefore the highest possible value of *eps* is 1 for the velocity magnitude and 2 for the pressure. The difference concerning the velocity in the axial slice is quite small, whereas the difference of the pressure in both the axial slice and on the surface varies significantly in the area underneath the constriction. This indicates that the solution with respect to the pressure as dependent variable is not grid independent in that area. In the comparison of both pharyngeal geometries in the second part of this section the pressure distribution is therefore omitted in the analysis. The simulations based on the pharyngeal model with MAA depicted in figure

4.10 show acceptable differences for both the velocity magnitude and the pressure for boundary condition type one.

In the case of boundary condition type two the variations in the velocity magnitude are acceptable small with and without MAA, as can be seen in figure 4.11 and 4.12. The pressure has high variations, but only in a small part of the domain, which is in the inlet area near the wall. Because the error is very small in the remaining domain, which is of more interest than the inlet area, the pressure distribution is still used for the comparison of the different geometries in the second part of this chapter. In each pharyngeal model the solutions for the four slices are compared for the two different grid sizes. The solutions are compared by their Reynolds number Re in each slice based on the mean kinematic viscosity and the hydraulic diameter computed by (2.29) and the mean velocity of that slice. Also the mean pressure of that slice is compared. The solutions are compared with respect to the error measure eps (3.18). The differences are in the most quite small for all variables, turbulence models, boundary conditions and both data types. In the most they are well below 0.05. There are only two exceptions in the case of boundary condition type one for the data without MAA and the simulations done without turbulence model for the mean pressure in slice 3 and 4. Those cases are excluded in the comparison of the simulations with and without MAA in section 4.2.2. The errors of the three examined quantities can be found in the appendix in tables 7.1-7.4.

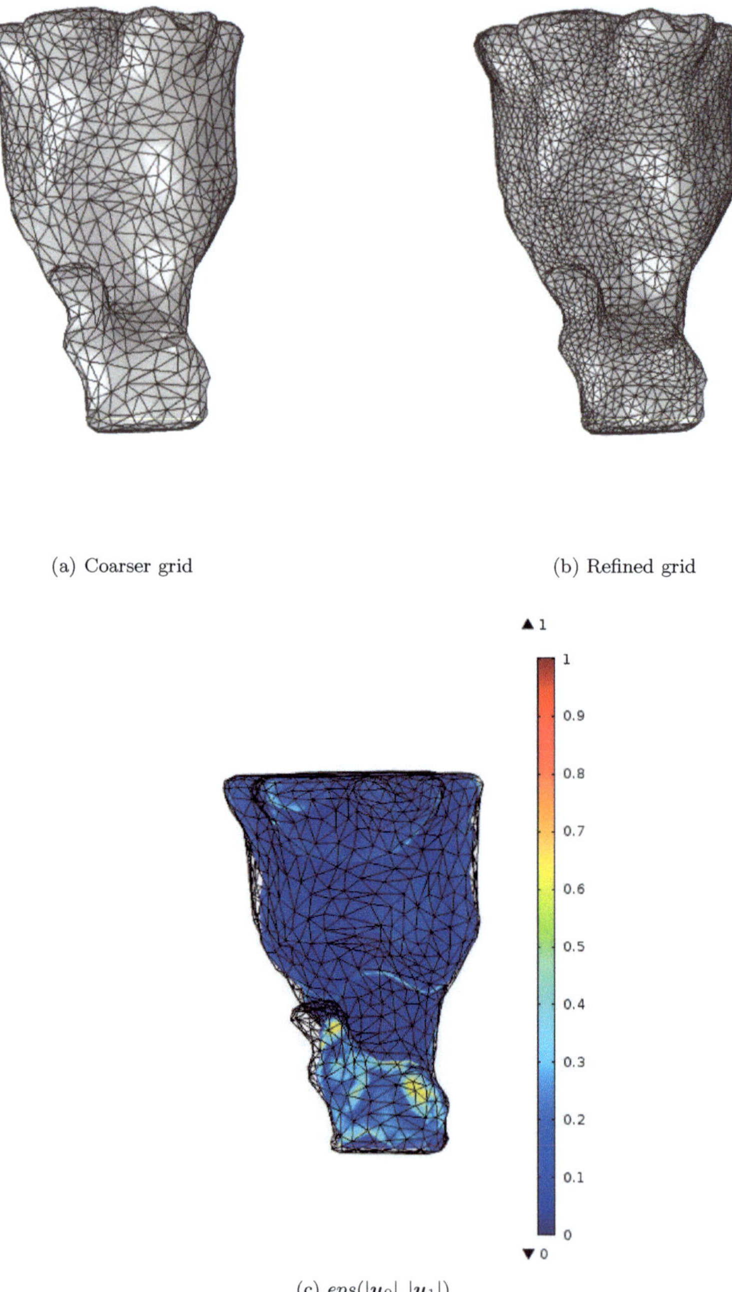

(a) Coarser grid

(b) Refined grid

(c) $eps(|\boldsymbol{u}_0|, |\boldsymbol{u}_1|)$

Figure 4.6: The error of the velocity magnitude of two solutions for the flow with boundary condition type one for the data without MAA on different grids is higher underneath the constriction area. A comparison with the overlay of the segmentations and the computed tomography datasets in figure 3.1 may be usable to relate the digitized models to the anatomical structures.

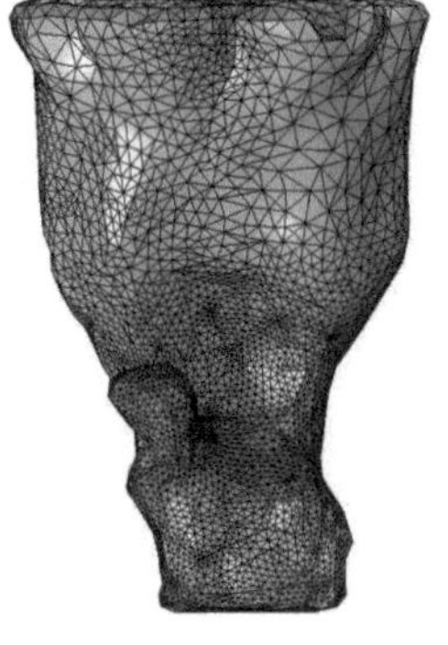 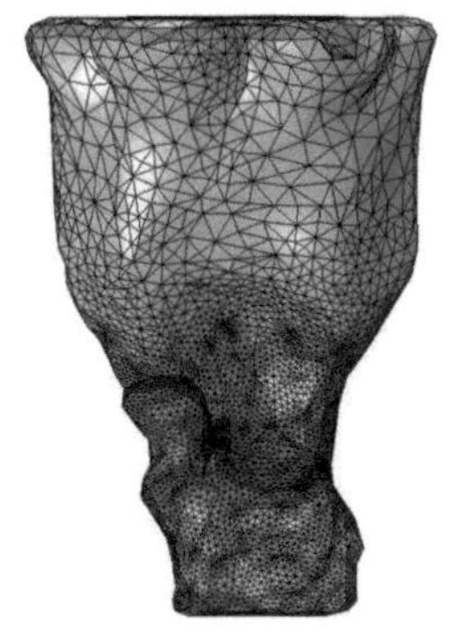 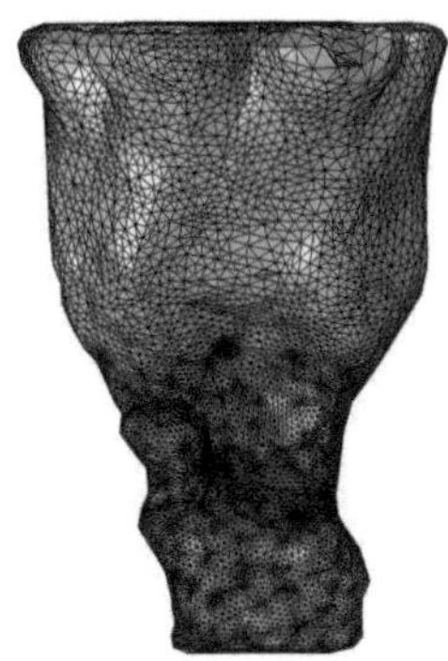

(a) Mesh with 198,882 elements   (b) Mesh with 231,207 elements   (c) Mesh with 534,589 elements

Figure 4.7: Adapted meshes for the data without MAA. The area of the constriction and underneath the constriction has a higher spatial resolution.

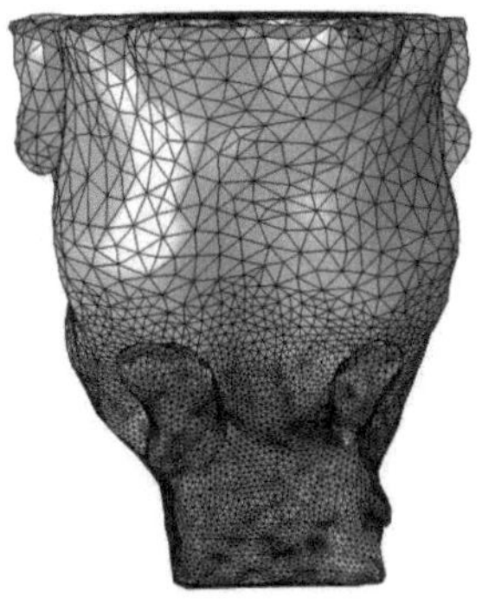 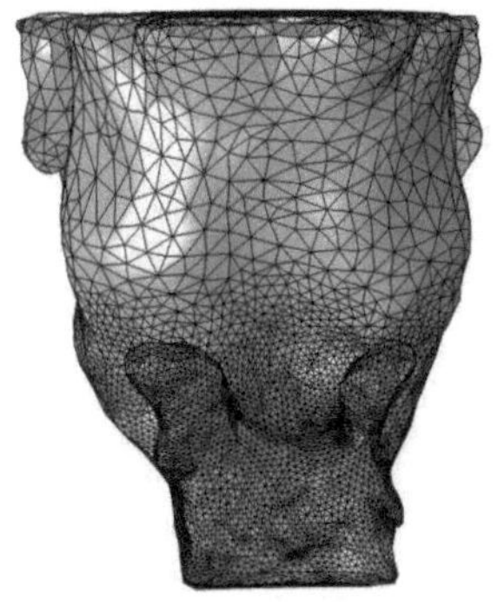 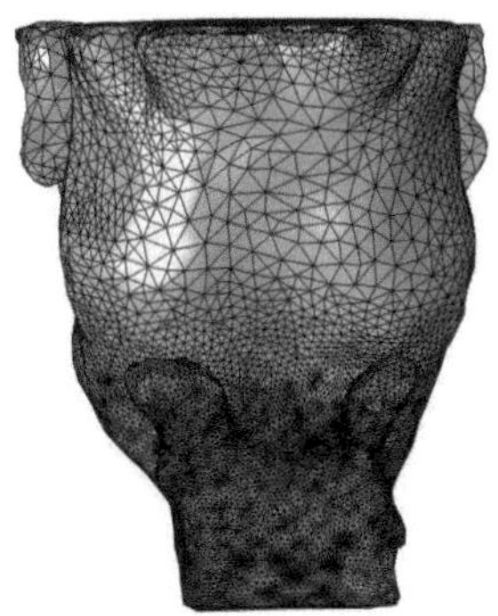

(a) Mesh with 238,440 elements   (b) Mesh with 373,803 elements   (c) Mesh with 587,375 elements

Figure 4.8: Adapted meshes for the data with MAA. The area of the constriction and underneath the constriction has a higher spatial resolution.

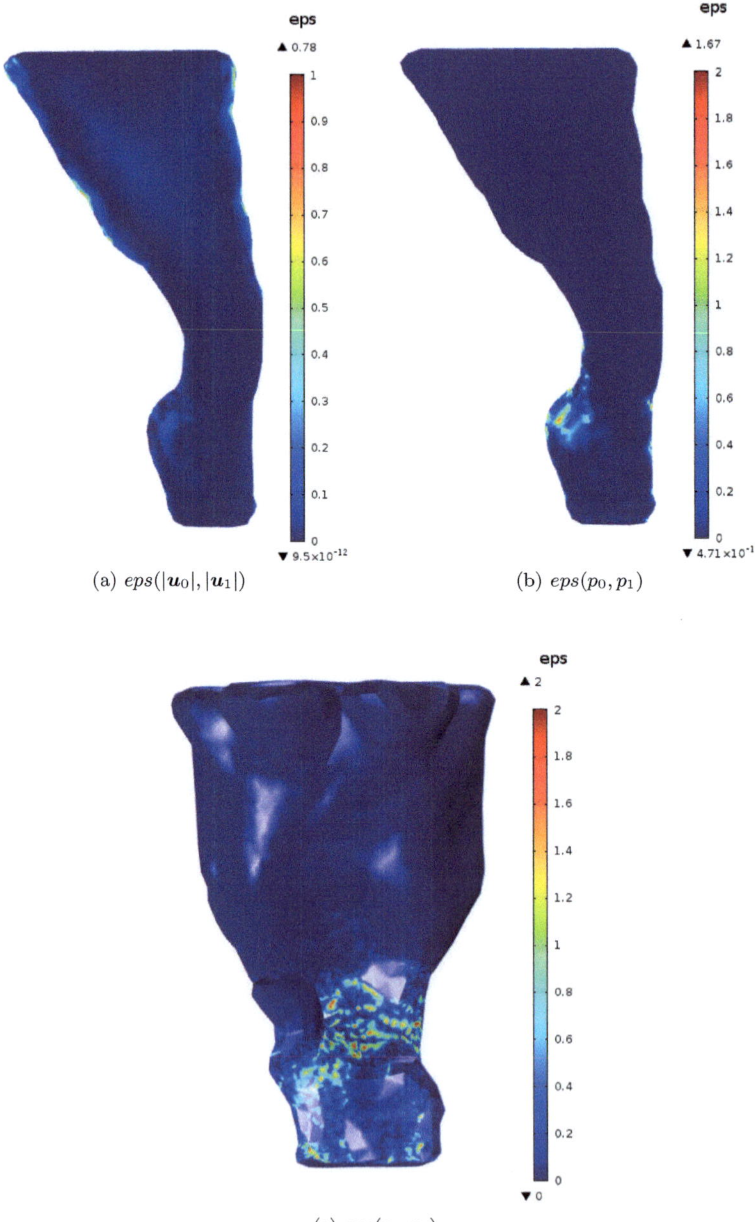

(a) $eps(|\boldsymbol{u}_0|, |\boldsymbol{u}_1|)$

(b) $eps(p_0, p_1)$

(c) $eps(p_0, p_1)$

Figure 4.9: Difference for the axial slice and the surface for the patient without MAA in the simulation with the $k - \omega$ turbulence model and boundary condition type one.

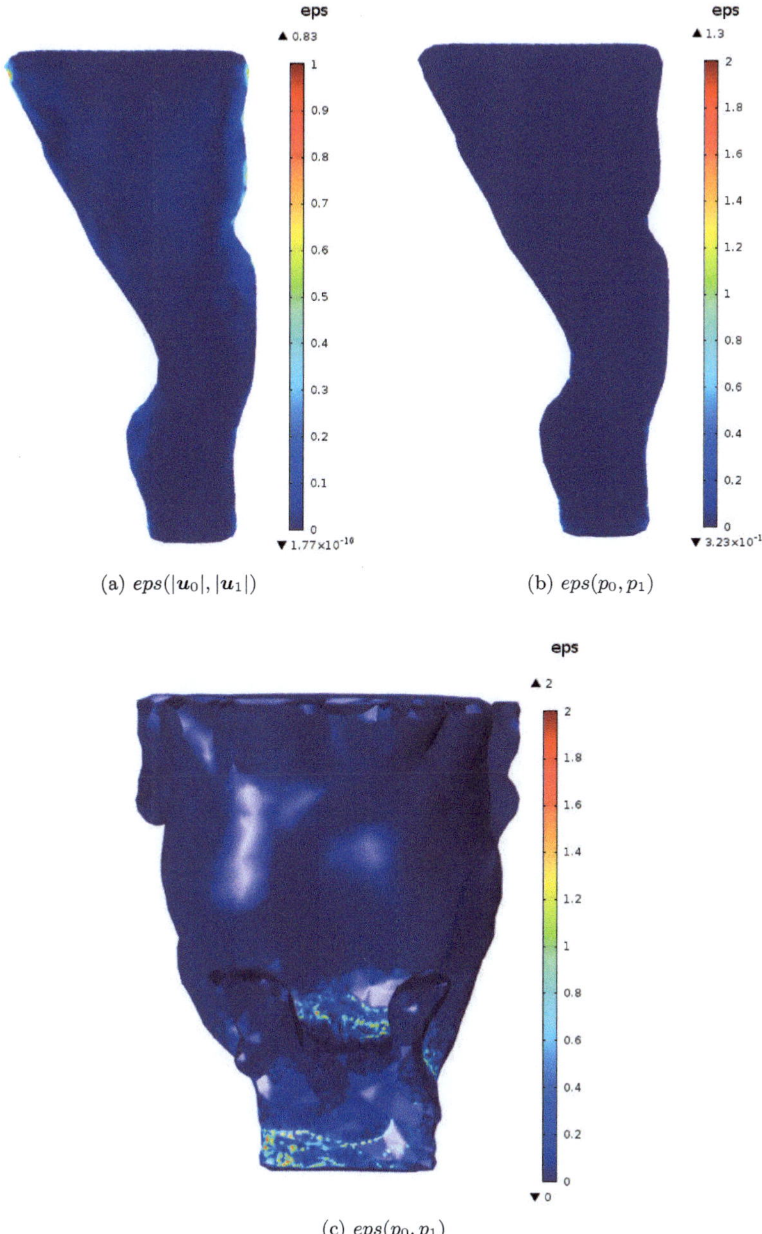

(a) $eps(|\boldsymbol{u}_0|, |\boldsymbol{u}_1|)$

(b) $eps(p_0, p_1)$

(c) $eps(p_0, p_1)$

Figure 4.10: Difference for the axial slice and the surface for the patient with MAA in the simulation with the $k - \omega$ turbulence model and boundary condition type one.

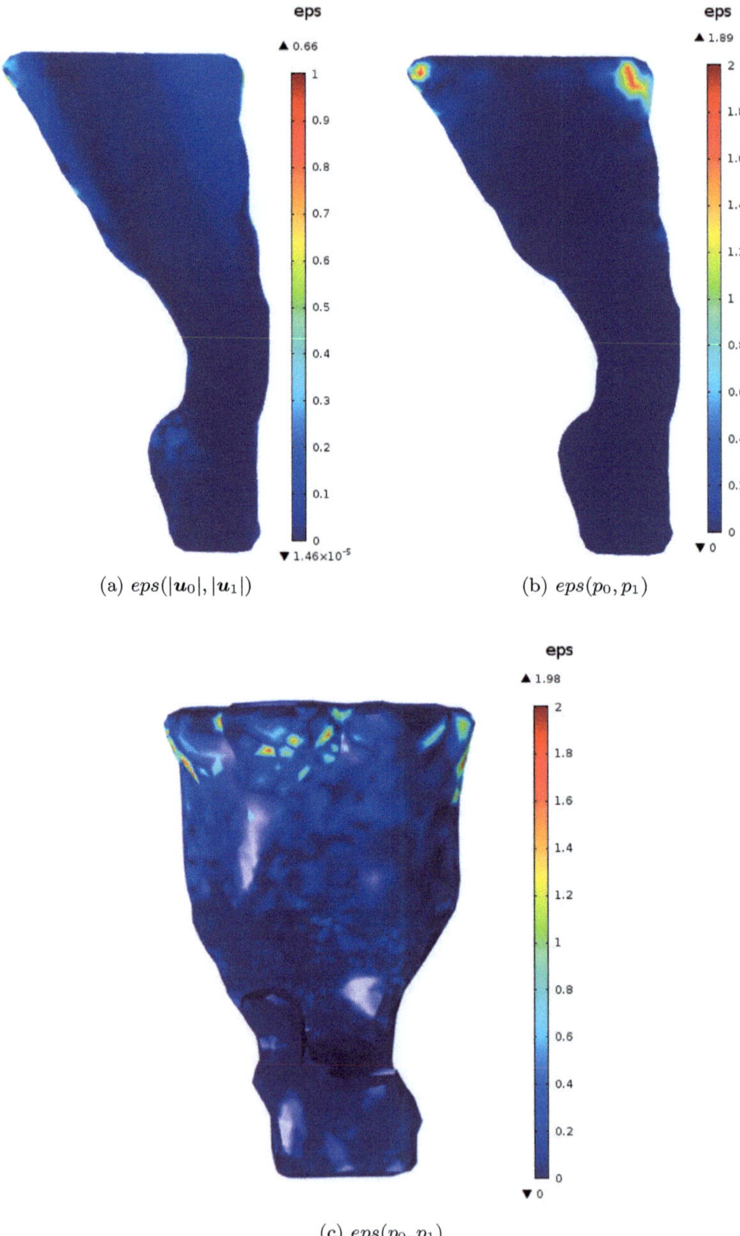

(a) $eps(|\boldsymbol{u}_0|, |\boldsymbol{u}_1|)$

(b) $eps(p_0, p_1)$

(c) $eps(p_0, p_1)$

Figure 4.11: Differences for the axial slice and the surface for the patient without MAA in the simulation with the $k - \omega$ turbulence model and boundary condition type one.

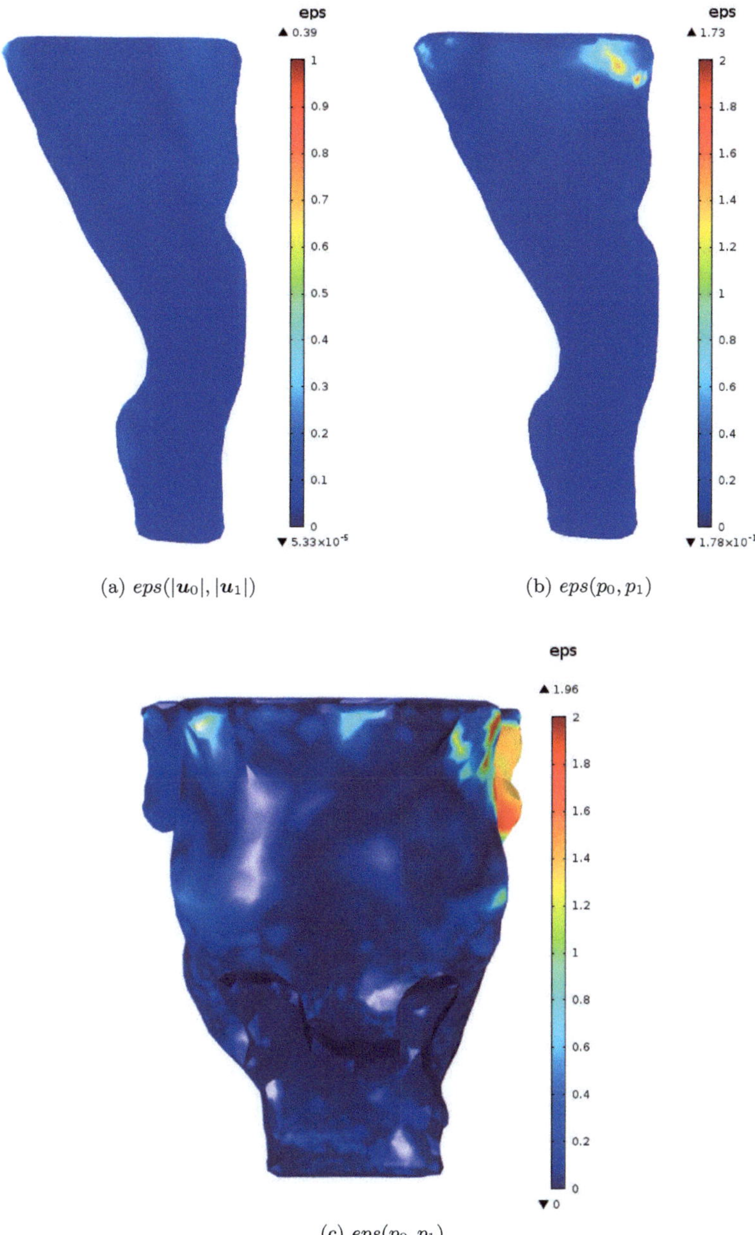

(a) $eps(|\boldsymbol{u}_0|, |\boldsymbol{u}_1|)$

(b) $eps(p_0, p_1)$

(c) $eps(p_0, p_1)$

Figure 4.12: Differences for the axial slice and the surface for the patient with MAA in the simulation with the $k - \omega$ turbulence model and boundary condition type one.

The turbulence parameters of the inflow stream are unknown and therefore estimated as described in the chapter 3. The influence of a 20 % variation to that quantities on the simulation results is tested for the data without MAA. As it shows up that the behavior is the same for both turbulence models and all variations of the different turbulence statistic parameters, the results are given in figure 4.13 only for the $k - \omega$ simulation with a 20 % increased turbulence intensity, remaining results can be found in the appendix from figure 7.6 to 7.16. The simulations with the variations are performed on the unrefined grid, the comparison is made with the simulations on the same meshes without variation on the parameters.

In figure 4.13 the difference of the simulation concerning the velocity magnitude and the pressure in the axial slice is given. For comparison reasons the difference resulting from the grid dependency studies with different mesh sizes are also depicted in the same figure. It can be seen that the differences resulting from the variation of the inlet parameters resemble the differences resulting from the usage of different grid sizes. This indicates that the differences do not reflect a changed flow behavior resulting from different inlet properties, but the sensitivity of a solution that is dependent on the grid on the variation of input parameters. To confirm this guess an additional solution is obtained with the variation of 20 % increased turbulence intensity on the solution for the pharyngeal lumen with MAA, because of the better grid independency of that solution. The result in figure 4.14 shows that the increase about 20% on the turbulence intensity does not change the solution.

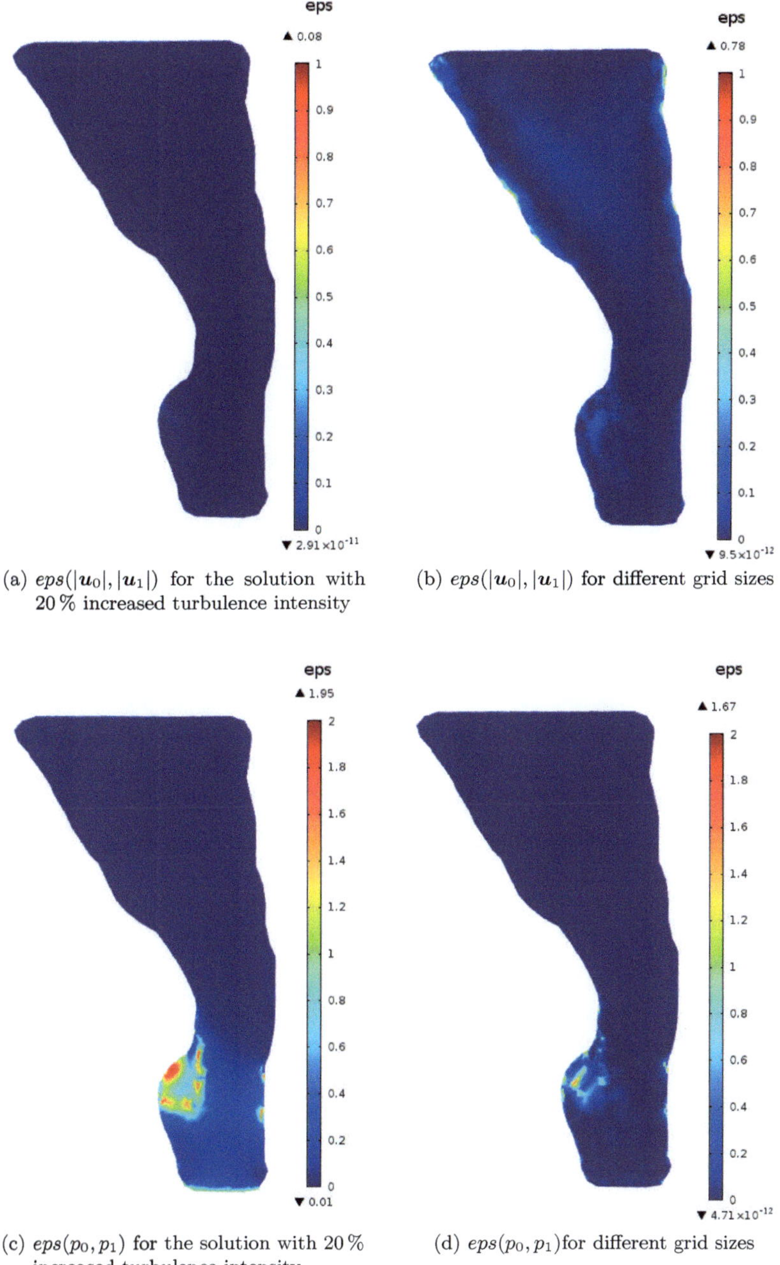

(a) $eps(|\boldsymbol{u}_0|, |\boldsymbol{u}_1|)$ for the solution with 20 % increased turbulence intensity

(b) $eps(|\boldsymbol{u}_0|, |\boldsymbol{u}_1|)$ for different grid sizes

(c) $eps(p_0, p_1)$ for the solution with 20 % increased turbulence intensity

(d) $eps(p_0, p_1)$ for different grid sizes

Figure 4.13: Differences for the axial slice for the patient without MAA in the simulation with the $k - \omega$ turbulence model and boundary condition type one and 20 % increased turbulence intensity at the inlet.

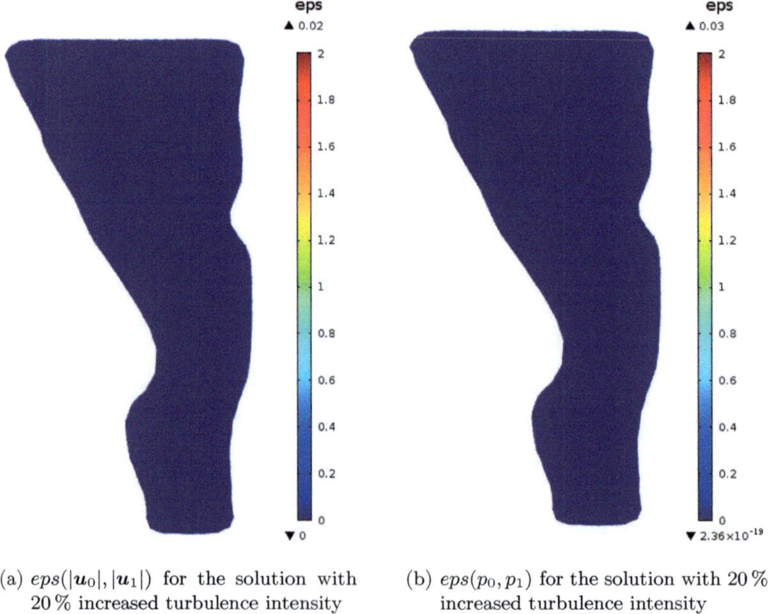

(a) $eps(|\boldsymbol{u}_0|, |\boldsymbol{u}_1|)$ for the solution with 20 % increased turbulence intensity

(b) $eps(p_0, p_1)$ for the solution with 20 % increased turbulence intensity

Figure 4.14: Differences for the axial slice for the patient with MAA in the simulation with the $k - \omega$ turbulence model and boundary condition type one and 20 % increased turbulence intensity at the inlet.

4.2.2 Comparison of patient data

Flow simulations are performed in the human pharynx of an OSAHS patient with and without MAA to examine the differences in the flow behavior. The simulation results concerning the flow velocity of both geometries and boundary type one are depicted in figure 4.15 for the simulation with Navier Stokes Equations, in figure 4.16 for the simulation using the $k - \epsilon$ turbulence model and in figure 4.17 using the $k - \omega$ turbulence model.

It shows up that the velocity magnitude in all three modeling types and both geometry types is enhanced after the constriction. So the constricted part leads to an increase of the flow velocity. But a reduction of nearly 50 % of the velocity magnitude after the constriction is achieved if the patient is wearing the MAA. A reduction of flow velocity directly after the constriction in the simulation with MAA in comparison to the simulation without MAA can also be seen in the results from the simulations using boundary type two for the $k - \epsilon$ model in figure 4.18 and for the $k - \omega$ model in figure 4.19, although the reduction is not as high as for boundary type one.

The comparison of the simulation results of the different geometries for boundary type two

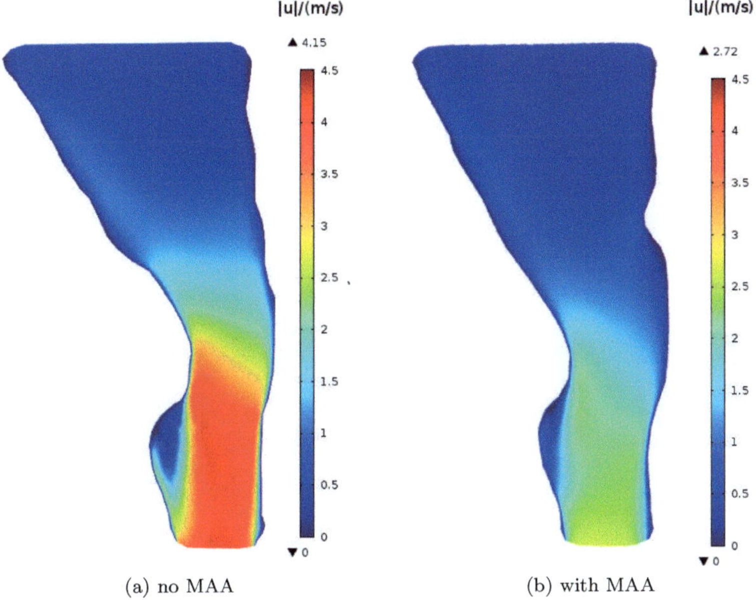

(a) no MAA   (b) with MAA

Figure 4.15: Visualization of the velocity magnitude in the axial slice in the simulation with Navier Stokes Equations and boundary conditions type one.

concerning the pressure distribution in the axial slice and on the surface given in figure 4.20 for the $k - \epsilon$ model and in figure 4.21 for the $k - \omega$ model show a reduction of the negative pressure in the area of the constriction and underneath, if the patient is wearing the MAA. The pressure in and underneath the constricted region in the pharynx without MAA is in the area of $-15\,\mathrm{Pa}$ to $-20\,\mathrm{Pa}$. In the geometry with MAA the pressure is between $-10\,\mathrm{Pa}$ and $-15\,\mathrm{Pa}$ in the same area.

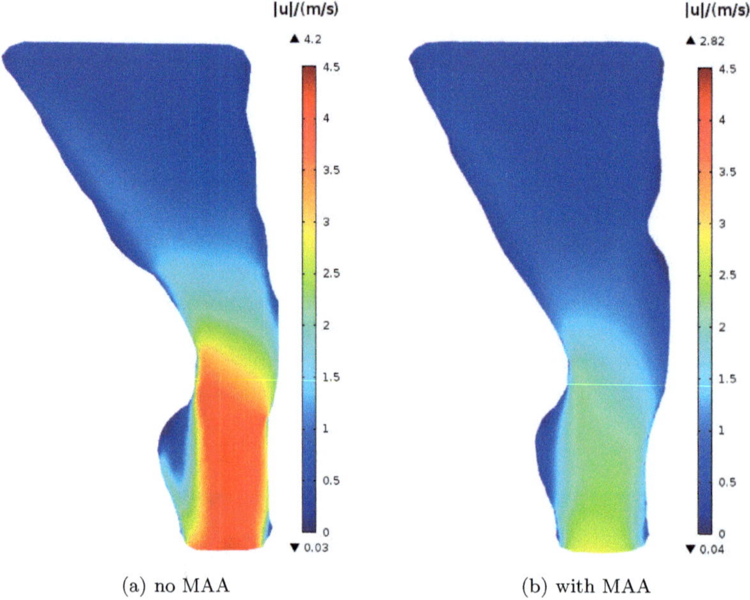

(a) no MAA (b) with MAA

Figure 4.16: Visualization of the velocity magnitude in the axial slice in the simulation with $k-\epsilon$ turbulence model and boundary conditions type one.

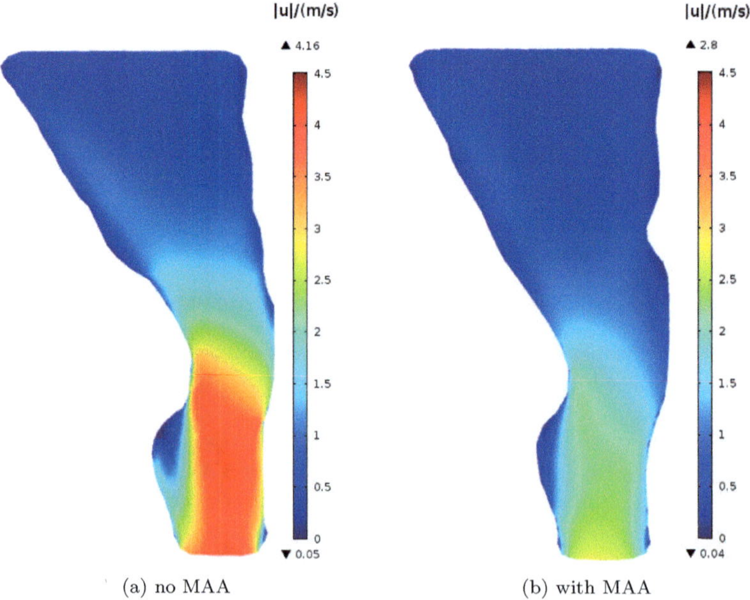

(a) no MAA (b) with MAA

Figure 4.17: Visualization of the velocity magnitude in the axial slice in the simulation with $k-\omega$ turbulence model and boundary conditions type one.

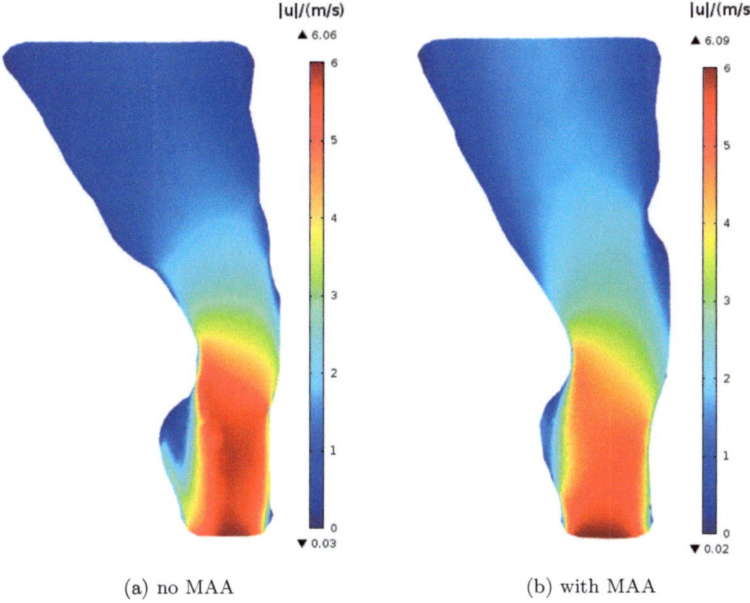

(a) no MAA
(b) with MAA

Figure 4.18: Visualization of the velocity magnitude in the axial slice in the simulation with $k-\epsilon$ turbulence model and boundary conditions type two.

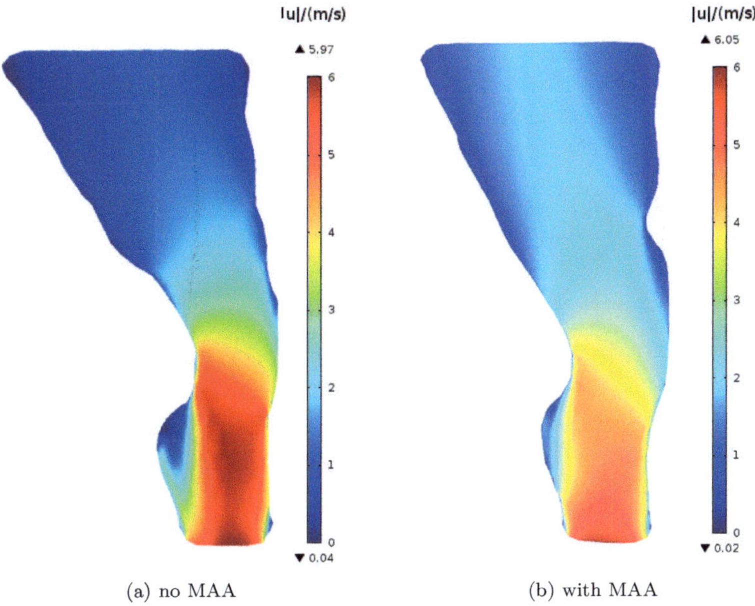

(a) no MAA
(b) with MAA

Figure 4.19: Visualization of the velocity magnitude in the axial slice in the simulation with $k-\omega$ turbulence model and boundary conditions type two.

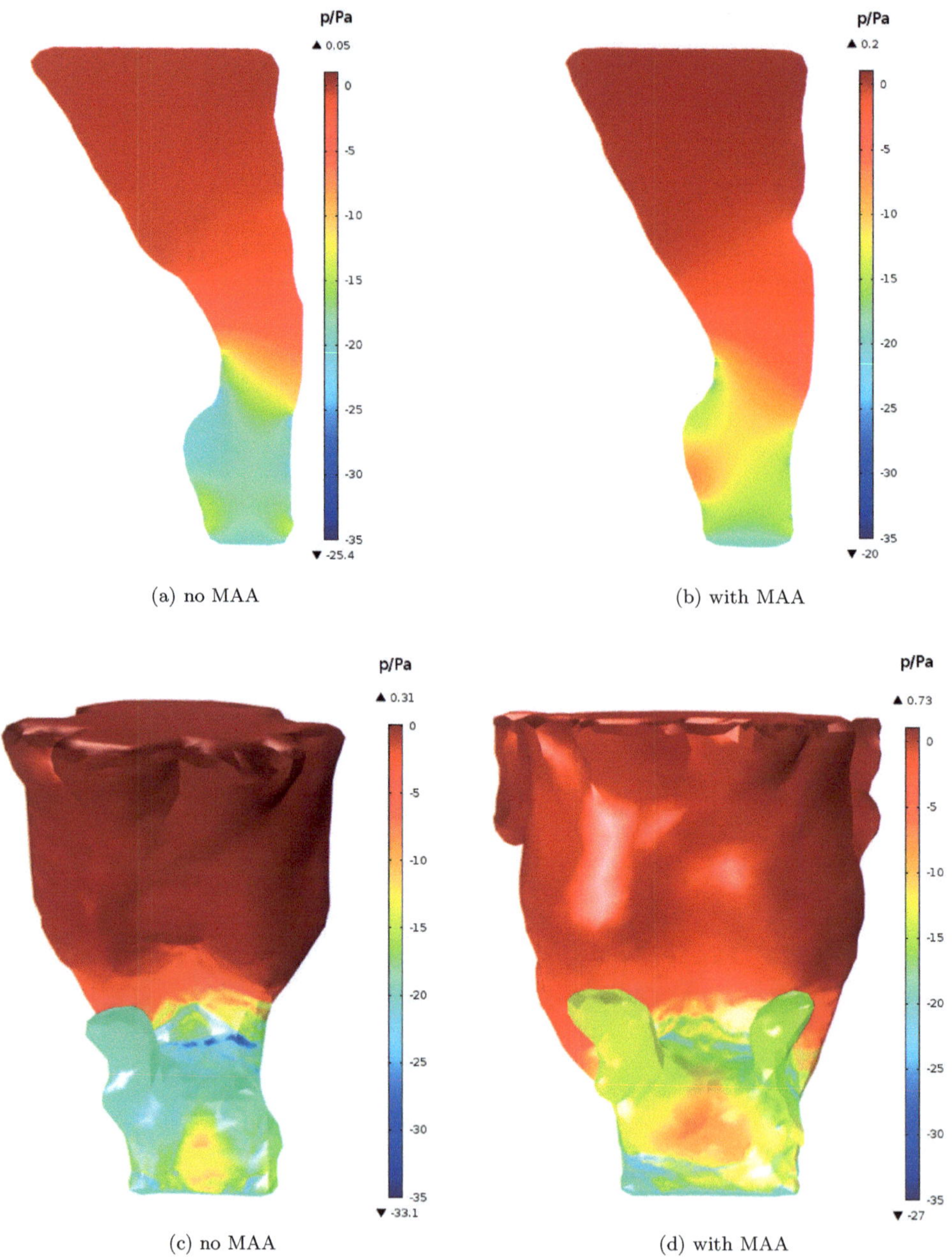

(a) no MAA

(b) with MAA

(c) no MAA

(d) with MAA

Figure 4.20: Visualization of the pressure in the axial slice and the surface in the simulation with $k - \epsilon$ turbulence model and boundary conditions type two.

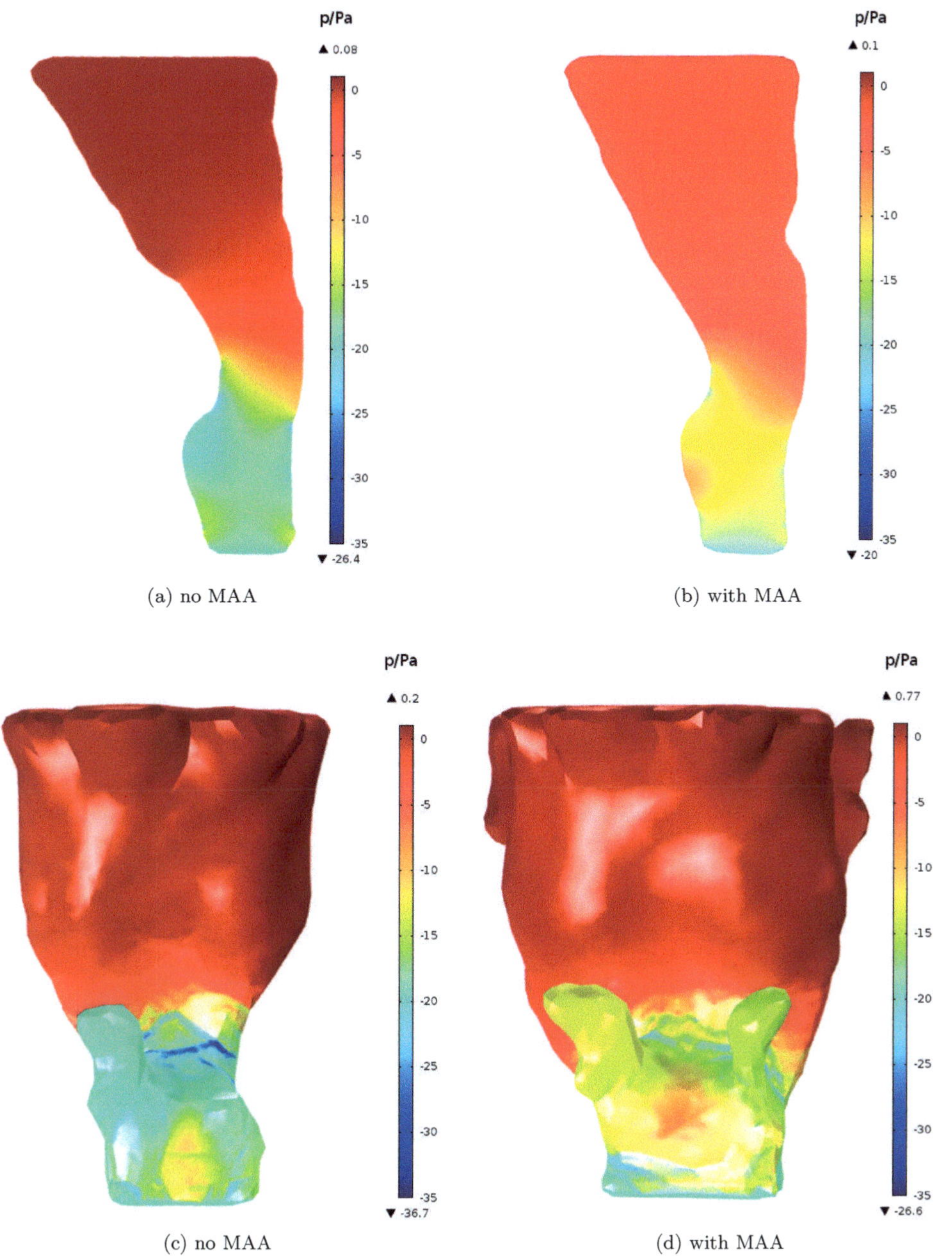

(a) no MAA

(b) with MAA

(c) no MAA

(d) with MAA

Figure 4.21: Visualization of the pressure in the axial slice and the surface in the simulation with $k - \omega$ turbulence model and boundary conditions type two.

The Reynolds numbers as well as the mean pressure in the four slices orthogonal to the axial direction of the pharynx are compared in figure 4.22 for boundary condition type one. The Reynolds number and the pressure are plotted against the distance from the inlet area, which is denoted with z^+. The graphs show three main points:

1. The Reynolds number is decreased in the presence of a MAA.

2. The pressure is lower in the presence of a MAA.

3. The results are nearly the same for all three modeling types.

In the case of boundary condition type two shown in figure 4.23 the third point can also be observed for the two turbulence models. But the first point, the reduction of the Reynolds number in the presence of a MAA is not the case for that boundary condition, although the velocity decreases too as earlier observed. The flow velocity reduction is not as high as in the case of boundary condition type one, and as the volume of the pharynx is enhanced in the presence of a MAA, the hydraulic diameter becomes also larger, which influences the Reynolds number. But a reduction of the magnitude of the pressure can be observed, as also seen in the visualization of the pressure distribution in the axial slice and on the surface.
The pressure for boundary type one is only in the positive regime and the highest pressure drop is at about 9 Pa, whereas the pressure for boundary condition type two is negative in the whole domain and the highest pressure drop is at about 18 Pa. These differences must result from the manner of prescribing the boundary conditions that had been 0 Pa pressure at the outlet for boundary condition type one and -20 Pa for boundary type two.
For the computation using boundary condition type two the finer grid is the same that is used as coarser grid for the computations of boundary condition type one. No simulation has been performed on the finer grid of boundary type one using boundary type two, because the simulation with boundary type two demands higher computational costs than for boundary condition type one, which is shown the number of iteration steps that are necessary for the computation. In table 4.1 the number of performed iteration steps are presented for the computation of the fluid flow for both turbulent models and both boundary condition types, that were necessary to derive the solution for the mesh with 231,207 elements for the data without MAA and 373,803 elements for the data with MAA. One iteration step means in this case one iteration of the segregated Newton iteration for the equation system solving for the velocity and the pressure and three Newton steps for the equation system solving for the turbulence variables k and ϵ and ω, respectively.

Table 4.1: Number of iteration steps for the solution of the different boundary condition types on the mesh with 231,207 elements for the pharynx without MAA and 373,803 elements for the pharynx with MAA. One iteration means one step of Newton iteration solving for the velocity and the pressure and three steps of Newton iterations solving for the turbulence variables.

		boundary condition type one	boundary condition type two
no MAA	$k - \epsilon$	35 iterations	57 iterations
	$k - \omega$	35 iterations	54 iterations
with MAA	$k - \epsilon$	31 iterations	68 iterations
	$k - \omega$	24 iterations	78 iterations

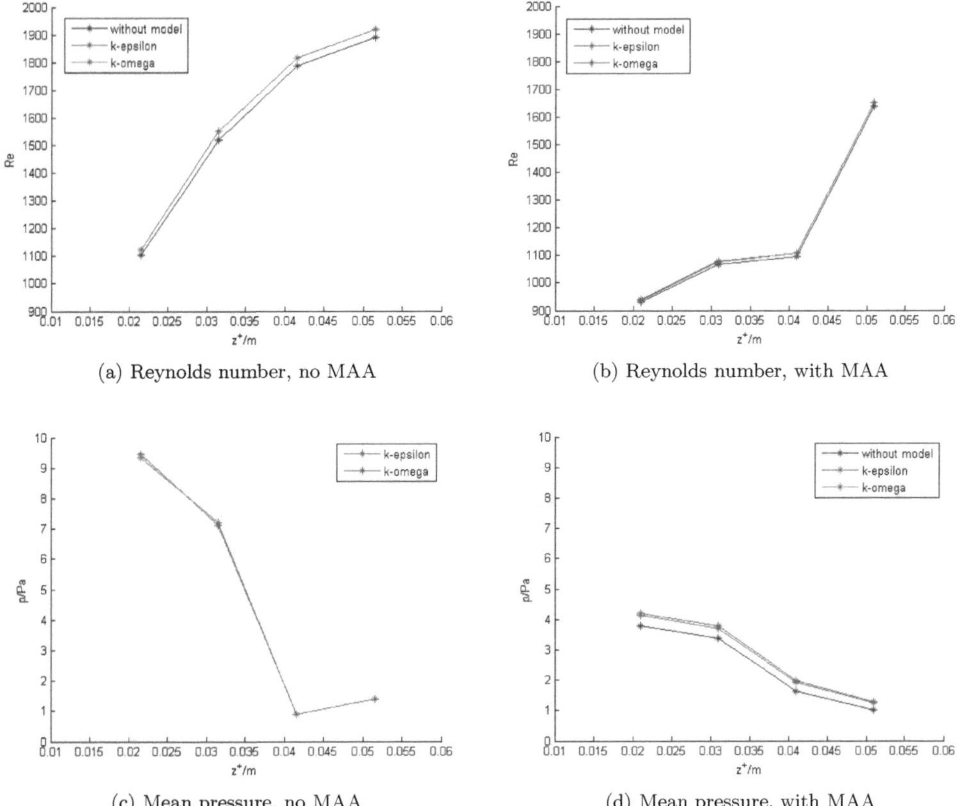

(a) Reynolds number, no MAA

(b) Reynolds number, with MAA

(c) Mean pressure, no MAA

(d) Mean pressure, with MAA

Figure 4.22: Reynolds number and mean pressure for the four slices in each pharyngeal model with and without MAA for the boundary condition type one. The position of the slices is described in distance from the inlet with z^+. The mean pressure for the solution without turbulence model is excluded from the analysis, because of its grid dependency.

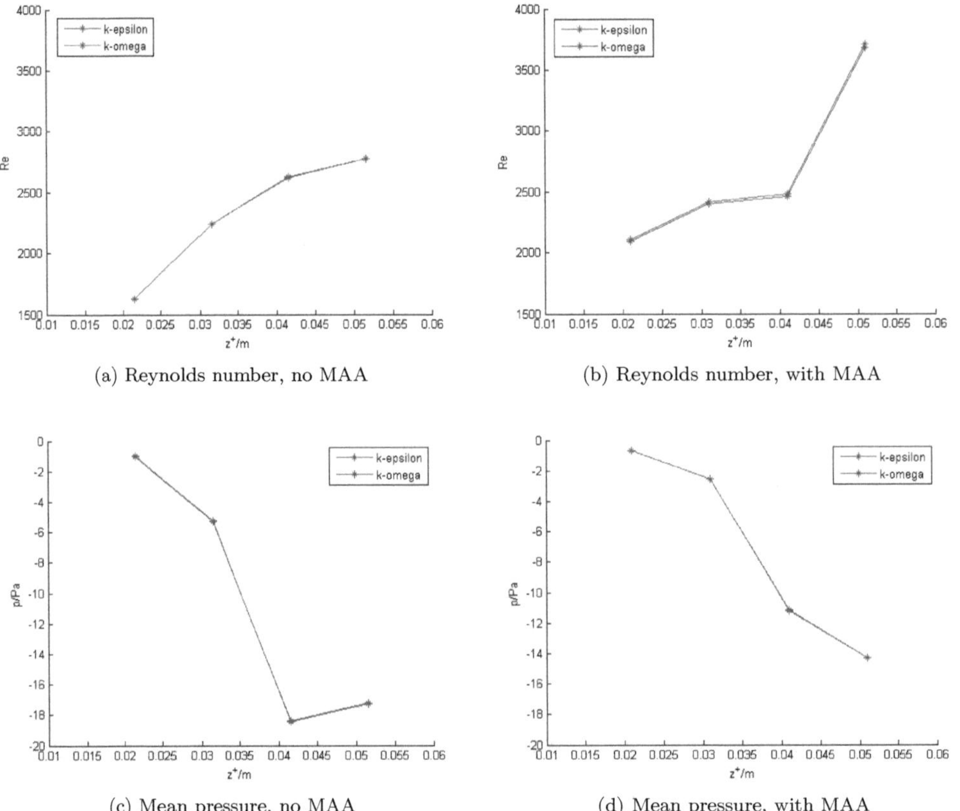

(a) Reynolds number, no MAA

(b) Reynolds number, with MAA

(c) Mean pressure, no MAA

(d) Mean pressure, with MAA

Figure 4.23: Reynolds number and mean pressure for the four slices in each pharyngeal model with and without MAA for the boundary condition type two. The position of the slices is described in distance from the inlet with z^+.

5 Discussion

Three parts of this work are discussed in the following: The agreement of the experimental measurements and the simulation on the arterial model, the comparison of simulation results in the pharyngeal anatomy with and without MAA and the reliability of that simulations.

5.1 Comparison to Measurement

Although the simulation on the finest grid shows a good match in most of the compared slices, the difference in slice $\Delta z = 2.5\, d$ is significant. This variance results from the asymmetry in the flow velocity profile. In the pipe no direction is distinguished from other directions, the flow should therefore exhibit a profile that oscillates symmetrically with respect to the centerline of the axial direction, which is also the case in the observed experimental setup by Ahmed and Giddens [2]. In the simulation on the coarsest mesh the profile shows preference to the lower side. The usage of that simulation result as initial solution for the following simulations may transfer this flow behavior on the following solutions. It is also possible that the flow is not fully developed in the time for which the solution on the finest grid had been computed and therefore the transition to a prefect symmetric oscillation is not accomplished. Because of the rotational invariance of the model geometry the preference of the lower side by the flow can only be explained by a dependency of the numerical solution on the direction. Despite that variation the simulation results are found to reflect the experiments by Ahmed and Giddens in a good manner, which validates the applicability of the COMSOL© simulation tool for fluid flow in pipes with a constriction area, to which generally spoken a pharynx with stenosis produced by the tongue belongs to.

It should also be mentioned that the turbulent oscillatory fluctuations can be reflected with a modeling type that is referred to as *laminar* in the COMSOL© environment. The denomination *laminar* for simulations without turbulence model can be quite misleading, because they use the Navier Stokes Equations which describe laminar as well as turbulent flow phenomena depending on the spatial and temporal resolution. If the resolution is not sufficiently dense, this may result in the solution failing to converge or converging to a wrong solution that misses the turbulent fluctuations.

5.2 Comparison of Patient Data

In the comparison of flow simulations in OSAHS patients the Reynolds number and the pressure are the most used parameters. Is is interesting to note that within this study the change of the Reynolds numbers resulting from a change of the flow velocity is a convincing parameter for the influence of the treatment with MAA in the case of boundary condition type one, the prescribed inlet velocity. This is different in the simulations with boundary type two, the prescribed pressure drop, where the Reynolds numbers even slightly increase in the presence of the MAA. But for the second boundary type the pressure shows a significant reaction on the treatment with the MAA. This shows that the extraction of physiological relevant parameters in fluid dynamics of OSAHS patients is strongly dependent on the choice of inlet and outlet boundary description.

The choice should therefore been physically realistic. Within this work the boundary condition type two describe a more realistic choice, because the prescribed pressure drop is a reflection of the inspiration process with the lung establishing a negative pressure. But this is also the boundary type that demands higher computational costs and may lead to convergence problems. Although two different turbulence models as well as simulations without turbulence modeling were examined no significant differences in the predicted flow phenomena could be observed in the different modeling techniques, besides that the simulation without turbulence model failed to converge in the case of boundary condition type two.

The Reynolds number in the simulations with boundary type one were in the area of laminar flow, but as Finlay et al. [28] assume, turbulence may there occur in a lower Reynolds number region because of the complex geometry of the human pharynx.

It should be remarked that it can not be concluded on a laminar flow just because a converged laminar solution can be obtained. The spatial resolution may not be as high enough to describe the turbulence of the flow. Certainty can only be derived in the comparison with experimental data. In the case of boundary type two no solution without turbulence model could be obtained. The reason therefor may be the occurring turbulence, which is indicated by Reynolds numbers in the laminar-to-turbulent transitional regime.

5.3 Reliability of the Models

Reliability of the simulations means the agreement of the performed simulations with the real flow within the patient's respiratory tract. Therefore the suitability of the digitized model and the grid dependency have to be regarded. The digitized model is the representation of the real human anatomy, approximations are inevitable in the process of achieving a digital model, but the model should be as accurate as possible. The approximation steps should be considered seriously. The first approximation to the real world is done with the cone beam CT image acquisition. The images have a low contrast which makes the distinction between pharyngeal volume and soft tissue more difficult. The segmentation is performed on the images with reduced resolution so that the voxels have a size of 1.2 mm in each spatial direction, which reduces the best possible spatial resolution of the digitized model to the same value. The surface triangulation of the segmentation uses flat triangular elements leading to a cornered digital model. A real human pharynx would not exhibit corners but smooth boundaries. A cornered geometry may enhance the development of turbulence and high pressure on artificial edges overestimating the real turbulence behavior.

The analysis of the grid dependency was performed within this work by comparing every variable using two grids with different numbers of mesh elements. The variables were used for the evaluation of the results if the difference is very small except of some parts in the computational domain, which were not regarded as determinant for the flow predictions like in the inlet region. The validation of each variable is a necessity, which can be concluded from the behavior of the flow simulations with boundary condition type one, where the axial velocity shows already quite small differences but the pressure differences are still higher. A grid dependency study that is performed regarding only one variable, or the average value of a variable, like for the computation of the Reynolds numbers can not be used to conclude on a grid independency of all variables in the whole domain. The process of validating the grid independency of only the interesting variables in the interesting part incorporates a serious problem: The equations used were of elliptical type, which means a variation of a variable anywhere in the domain can influence every other part of the solution. Hence, even if the variations of a variable in a selected area are very low, it can not be concluded that the simulated solution is close to the correct solution of the modeling equations as the low error indicates. To achieve certainty a grid dependency study would be necessary that results in an acceptable low error for all appearing variables in the whole computational domain. That was not possible within this work because of high computational costs. Computation times were already in the area of 20 hours and more on a system with 48 2.1 GHz processors and 128 GB RAM.

Because of the high computational costs the grids for the simulations with boundary condition type two did not change in size as much as for boundary condition type one. For the simulation without MAA the grid sizes in the simulations differ about 10 %. The results of the grid independency study may therefore look superior.

6 Conclusion and Outlook

Within this work it could be shown that the airflow in a human pharynx of an OSAHS patient with and without medical treatment in terms of a mandibular repositioning device differs from each other with respect to the flow velocity and the occurring pressures. The results agree with results by other authors, which may give the possibility to evaluate the severity of illness based on fluid simulations. If the possibility would exist to achieve a digitized representation of the geometry after an upper airway surgery by in-silico simulations of the soft tissue deformations, it could even be possible to evaluate surgery results before the treatment has been carried out, which would be a great advantage in individual patient therapy planning and could prevent unnecessary surgical interventions.

Within this work it has also been shown that for the analysis of parameters with physiological relevance the choice of boundary conditions is demanding. Depending on the choice of boundary conditions the Reynolds numbers and pressures lead to simulations in different clarity about the success of the treatment. A further step concerning this point could be the analysis of a larger number of patient datasets, taking information about the individual severity of the illness into account. With these information the significance of simulated values like the pressure distribution in the patient's pharynx could be evaluated.

The usage of digitized pharynx models that are more accurate could also lead to an enhancement in the validity of the flow simulations. The accuracy of the digitized models could be increased for example in using medical data with a higher contrast and higher spatial resolution and data with a better representation of soft tissue like MRT data. A more realistic representation of the surface triangulation could be achieved by using curved elements.

The validation of numerical simulations with experimental data of an artery stenosis showed good agreement, despite a preference of the resulting flow stream to one direction. Because of the rotational invariance of the geometry the flow stream should not prefer one direction. The reason therefore must lie in some numerical orientation dependency in the solution process, maybe in the solver algorithms or the preconditioning or stabilization parts. In order to find the reason for this asymmetry, it would be necessary to use self-made implementations instead of the simulation package COMSOL© to have a closer look at the implemented code.

Within this work no differences in the predictions of the two applied turbulence models as well as the simulation with the Navier Stokes Equations, where it was applicable, could be observed. The next step would be to validate the simulation results with experimental data. The realization of a hardware model based on digitized models is necessary. Zélicourt et al. [19] described a process to transform complex digital geometries into replicas made of optical transparent materials in which fluid flow can be examined using Particle Image Velocimetry (PIV). They used a three-dimensional stereolithographic printing technique with transparent resins, which enables the possibility to transform even very complex geometries in experimental setups accessible for optical examinations. Zélicourt et al. demonstrated the described method by comparing CFD simulations with experimental data resulting from the application of the printing technique on a cavopulmonary connection morphology.

This procedure could be used to derive experimental data of the flow field in anatomical correct human pharynx of living patients as well. Additionally the hardware model may also be usable to derive information about the pressure distribution, which is also a necessary demand in validating the agreement of experiments and simulation results.

7 Appendix

Table 7.1: Difference with respect to (3.18) for the Reynolds number Re and the mean pressure p_{mean} in four different slices for the solution in the two different grids for the patient's data without MAA and boundary condition type one. For shortening reasons $eps(\psi_0, \psi_1)$ is denoted with $eps(\psi)$.

slice	Navier Stokes Equations		$k - \epsilon$		$k - \omega$	
	$eps(Re)$	$eps(p_{\mathrm{mean}})$	$eps(Re)$	$eps(p_{\mathrm{mean}})$	$eps(Re)$	$eps(p_{\mathrm{mean}})$
1	0.012	0.043	0.001	0.013	0.001	0.015
2	0.012	0.049	0.000	0.018	0.000	0.010
3	0.011	0.235	0.000	0.003	0.000	0.005
4	0.011	0.133	0.000	0.023	0.000	0.019

Table 7.2: Difference with respect to (3.18) for the Reynolds number Re and the mean pressure p_{mean} in four different slices for the solution in the two different grids for the patient's data without MAA and boundary condition type two. For shortening reasons $eps(\psi_0, \psi_1)$ is denoted with $eps(\psi)$.

slice	$k - \epsilon$		$k - \omega$	
	$eps(Re)$	$eps(p_{\mathrm{mean}})$	$eps(Re)$	$eps(p_{\mathrm{mean}})$
1	0.004	0.013	0.005	0.015
2	0.005	0.003	0.006	0.004
3	0.005	0.004	0.006	0.003
4	0.005	0.007	0.006	0.005

Table 7.3: Difference with respect to (3.18) for the Reynolds number Re and the mean pressure p_{mean} in four different slices for the solution in the two different grids for the patient's data with MAA and boundary condition type one. For shortening reasons $eps(\psi_0, \psi_1)$ is denoted with $eps(\psi)$.

slice	Navier Stokes Equations		$k - \epsilon$		$k - \omega$	
	$eps(Re)$	$eps(p_{\mathrm{mean}})$	$eps(Re)$	$eps(p_{\mathrm{mean}})$	$eps(Re)$	$eps(p_{\mathrm{mean}})$
1	0.005	0.012	0.003	0.013	0.001	0.010
2	0.005	0.013	0.001	0.012	0.000	0.011
3	0.004	0.014	0.000	0.011	0.000	0.012
4	0.005	0.024	0.000	0.002	0.000	0.008

Table 7.4: Difference with respect to (3.18) for the Reynolds number Re and the mean pressure p_{mean} in four different slices for the solution in the two different grids for the patient's data with MAA and boundary condition type two. For shortening reasons $eps(\psi_0, \psi_1)$ is denoted with $eps(\psi)$.

slice	$k - \epsilon$		$k - \omega$	
	$eps(Re)$	$eps(p_{\mathrm{mean}})$	$eps(Re)$	$eps(p_{\mathrm{mean}})$
1	0.007	0.081	0.005	0.011
2	0.002	0.033	0.005	0.002
3	0.003	0.002	0.005	0.005
4	0.003	0.001	0.005	0.006

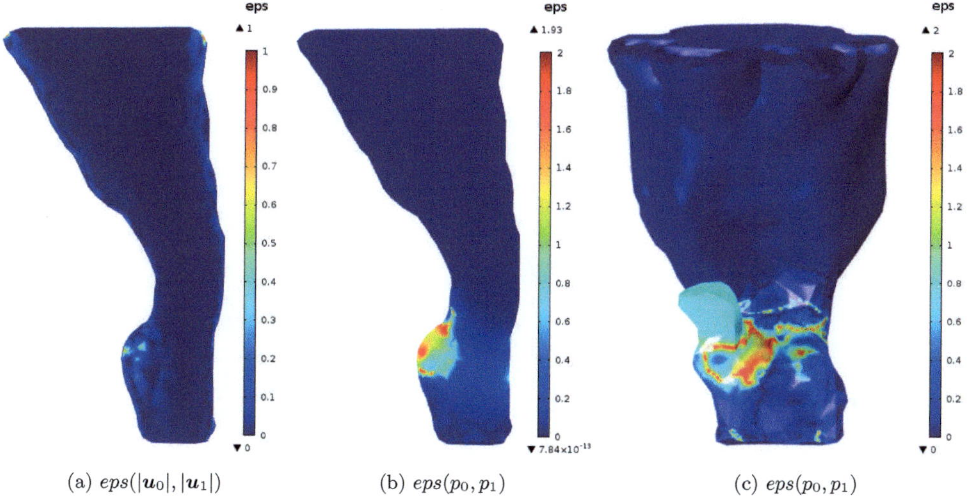

(a) $eps(|\boldsymbol{u}_0|, |\boldsymbol{u}_1|)$ (b) $eps(p_0, p_1)$ (c) $eps(p_0, p_1)$

Figure 7.1: Differences for the axial slice and the surface for the patient without MAA in the simulation with Navier Stokes Equations and boundary condition type one.

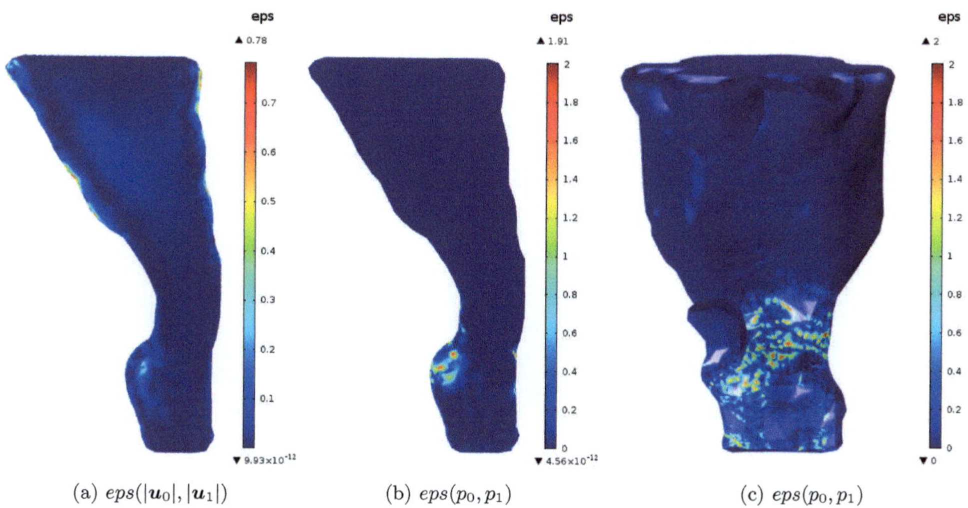

(a) $eps(|\boldsymbol{u}_0|, |\boldsymbol{u}_1|)$ (b) $eps(p_0, p_1)$ (c) $eps(p_0, p_1)$

Figure 7.2: Differences for the axial slice and the surface for the patient without MAA in the simulation with the $k - \epsilon$ turbulence model and boundary condition type one.

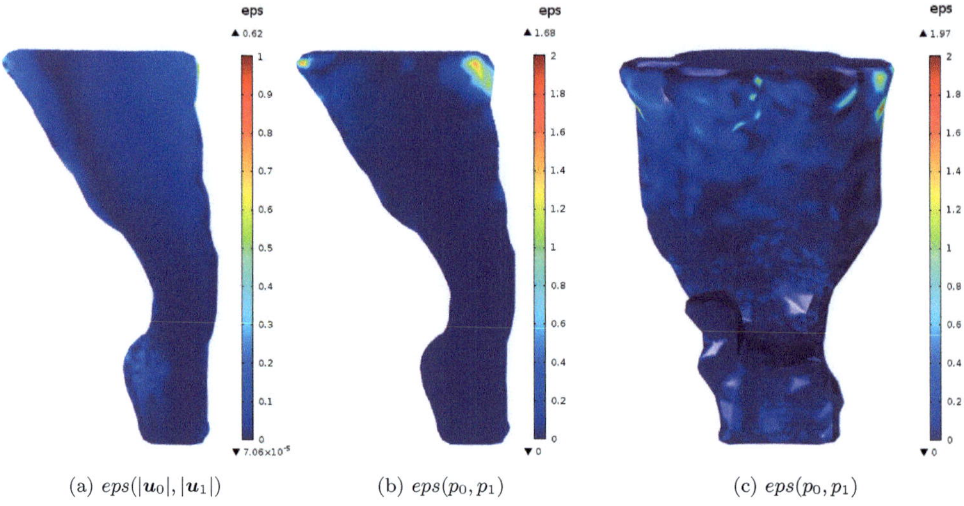

(a) $eps(|\boldsymbol{u}_0|, |\boldsymbol{u}_1|)$ (b) $eps(p_0, p_1)$ (c) $eps(p_0, p_1)$

Figure 7.3: Difference for the axial slice and the surface for the patient without MAA in the simulation with the $k - \epsilon$ turbulence model and boundary condition type two.

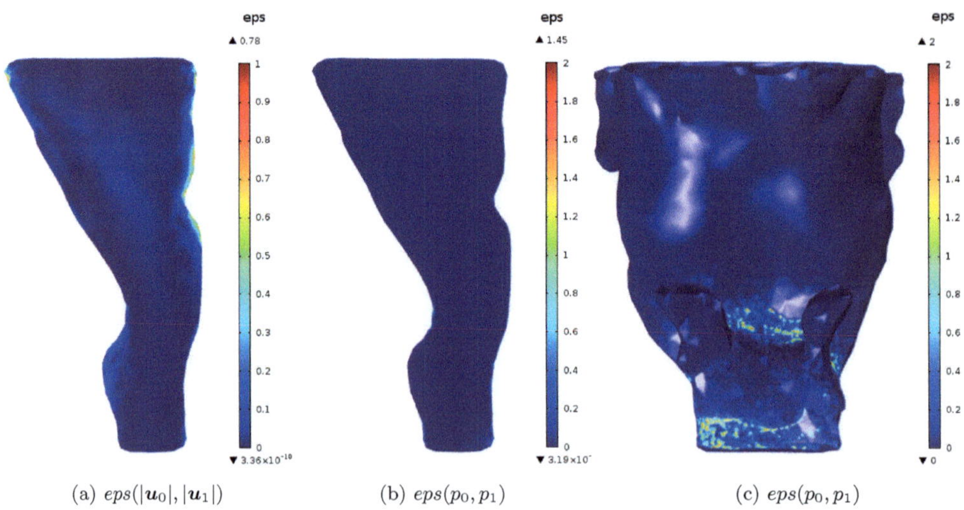

(a) $eps(|\boldsymbol{u}_0|, |\boldsymbol{u}_1|)$ (b) $eps(p_0, p_1)$ (c) $eps(p_0, p_1)$

Figure 7.4: Differences for the axial slice and the surface for the patient with MAA in the simulation with the $k - \epsilon$ turbulence model and boundary condition type one.

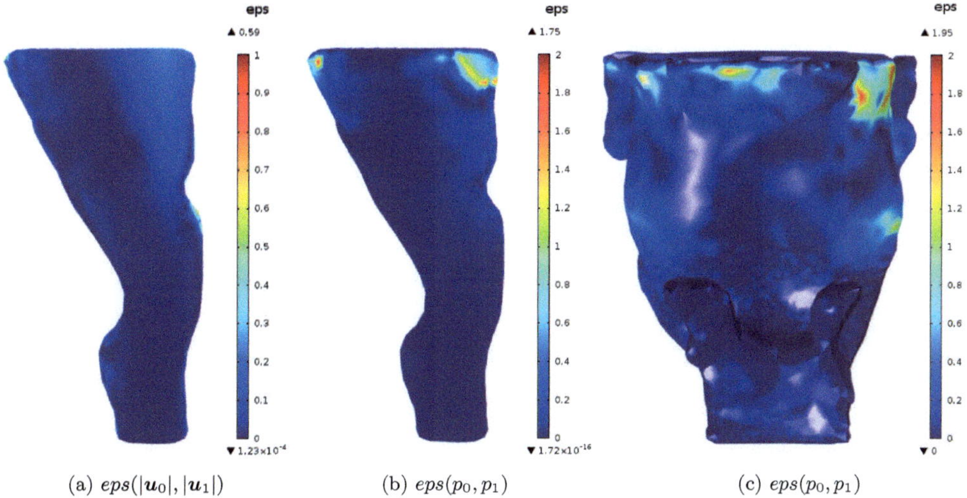

(a) $eps(|\boldsymbol{u}_0|, |\boldsymbol{u}_1|)$ (b) $eps(p_0, p_1)$ (c) $eps(p_0, p_1)$

Figure 7.5: Difference for the axial slice and the surface for the patient with MAA in the simulation with the $k - \epsilon$ turbulence model and boundary condition type two.

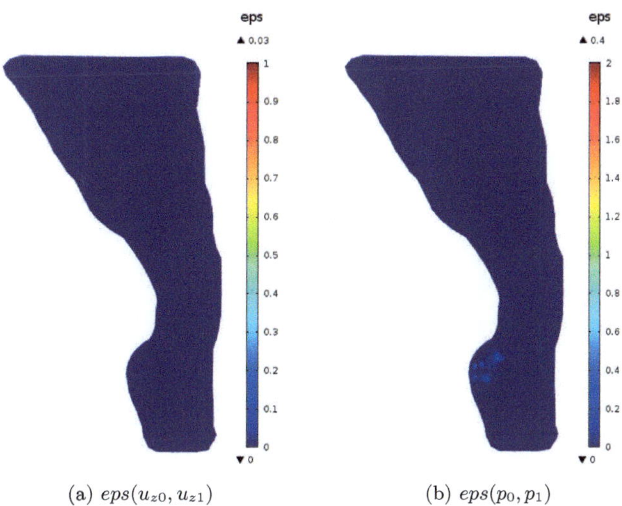

(a) $eps(u_{z0}, u_{z1})$ (b) $eps(p_0, p_1)$

Figure 7.6: Difference for the axial slice for the patient without MAA in the simulation with the $k - \epsilon$ turbulence model and boundary condition type one and 20 % increased turbulence intensity at the inlet.

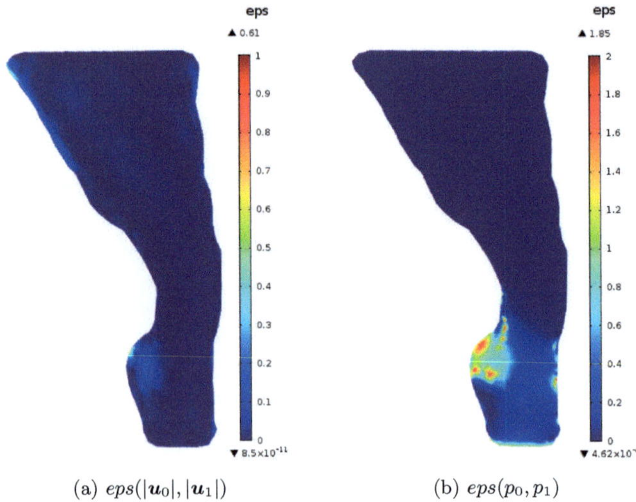

(a) $eps(|\boldsymbol{u}_0|, |\boldsymbol{u}_1|)$ (b) $eps(p_0, p_1)$

Figure 7.7: Difference for the axial slice for the patient without MAA in the simulation with the $k - \omega$ turbulence model and boundary condition type one and 20 % decreased turbulence intensity at the inlet.

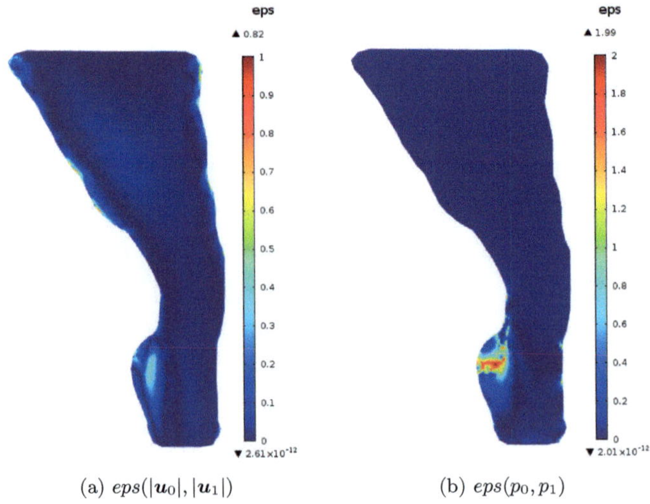

(a) $eps(|\boldsymbol{u}_0|, |\boldsymbol{u}_1|)$ (b) $eps(p_0, p_1)$

Figure 7.8: Difference for the axial slice for the patient without MAA in the simulation with the $k - \epsilon$ turbulence model and boundary condition type one and 20 % decreased turbulence intensity at the inlet.

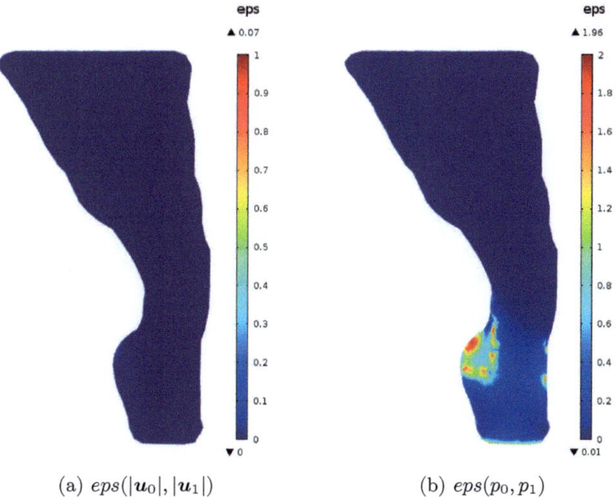

(a) $eps(|\boldsymbol{u}_0|, |\boldsymbol{u}_1|)$ (b) $eps(p_0, p_1)$

Figure 7.9: Difference for the axial slice for the patient without MAA in the simulation with the $k - \omega$ turbulence model and boundary condition type one and 20 % increased turbulence length scale at the inlet.

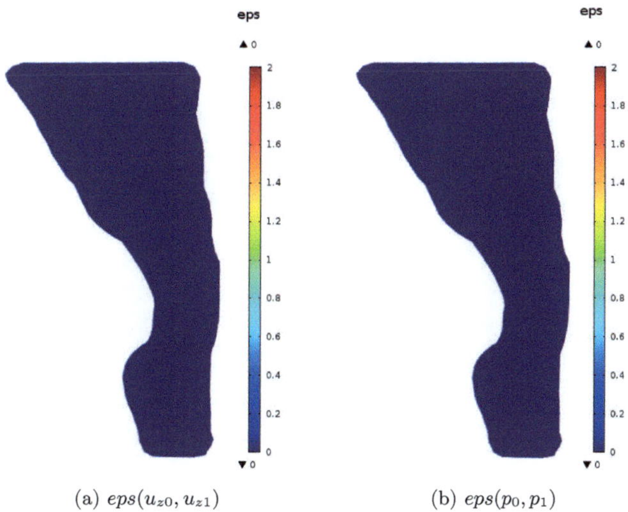

(a) $eps(u_{z0}, u_{z1})$ (b) $eps(p_0, p_1)$

Figure 7.10: Difference for the axial slice for the patient without MAA in the simulation with the $k - \epsilon$ turbulence model and boundary condition type one and 20 % increased turbulence length scale at the inlet.

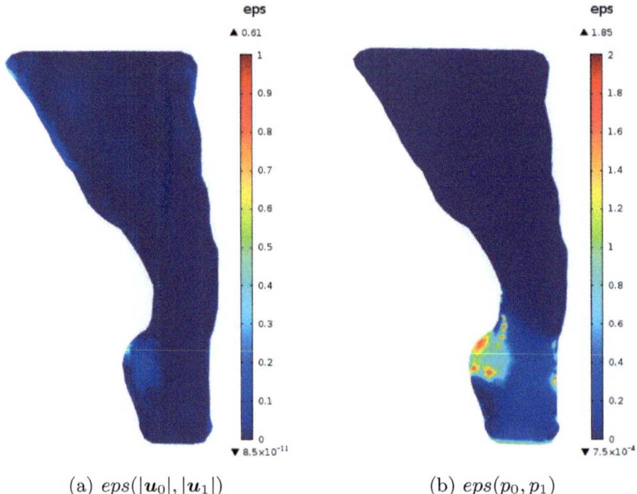

(a) $eps(|\boldsymbol{u}_0|, |\boldsymbol{u}_1|)$ (b) $eps(p_0, p_1)$

Figure 7.11: Difference for the axial slice for the patient without MAA in the simulation with the $k - \omega$ turbulence model and boundary condition type one and $20\,\%$ decreased turbulence length scale at the inlet.

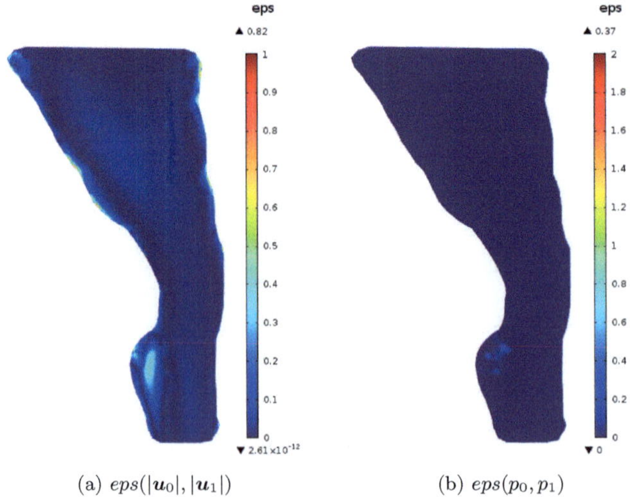

(a) $eps(|\boldsymbol{u}_0|, |\boldsymbol{u}_1|)$ (b) $eps(p_0, p_1)$

Figure 7.12: Difference for the axial slice for the patient without MAA in the simulation with the $k - \epsilon$ turbulence model and boundary condition type one and $20\,\%$ decreased turbulence length scale at the inlet.

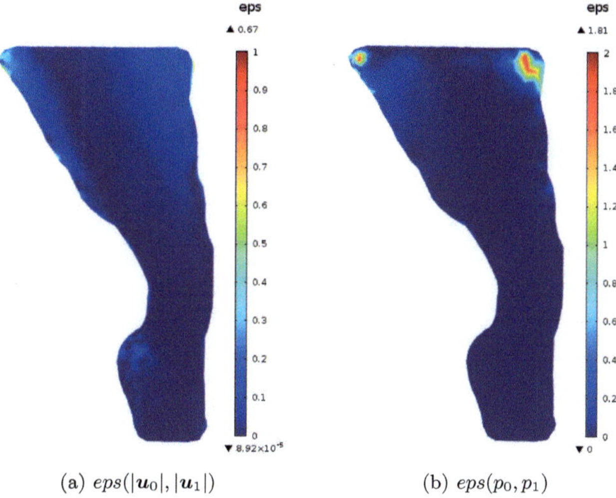

(a) $eps(|\boldsymbol{u}_0|, |\boldsymbol{u}_1|)$ (b) $eps(p_0, p_1)$

Figure 7.13: Difference for the axial slice for the patient without MAA in the simulation with the $k - \omega$ turbulence model and boundary condition type two and 20 % increased reference velocity scale at the inlet.

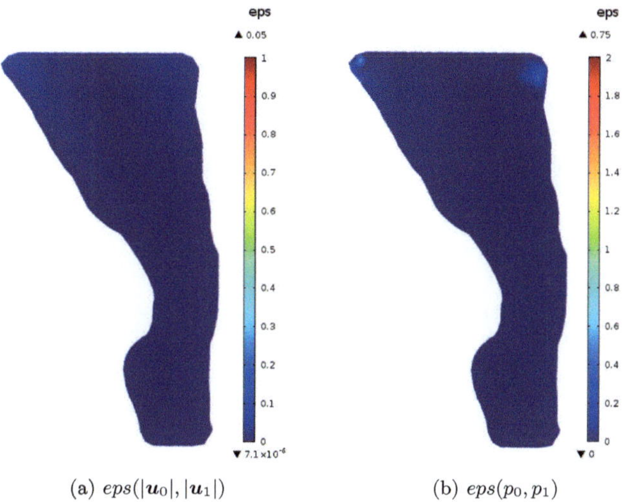

(a) $eps(|\boldsymbol{u}_0|, |\boldsymbol{u}_1|)$ (b) $eps(p_0, p_1)$

Figure 7.14: Difference for the axial slice for the patient without MAA in the simulation with the $k - \epsilon$ turbulence model and boundary condition type two and 20 % increased reference velocity scale at the inlet.

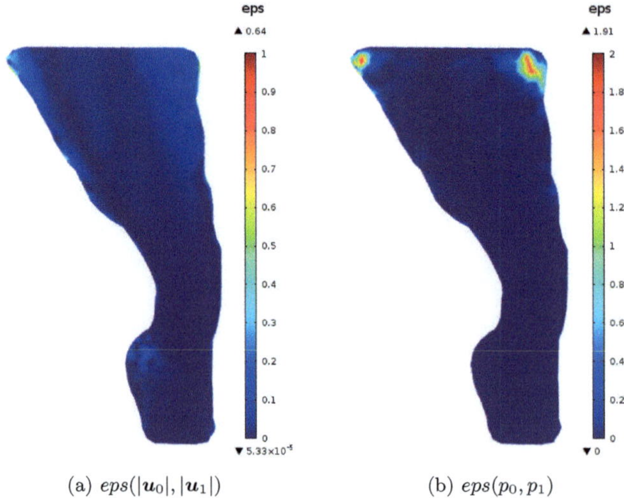

(a) $eps(|\boldsymbol{u}_0|, |\boldsymbol{u}_1|)$ (b) $eps(p_0, p_1)$

Figure 7.15: Difference for the axial slice for the patient without MAA in the simulation with the $k - \omega$ turbulence model and boundary condition type two and 20 % decreased reference velocity scale at the inlet.

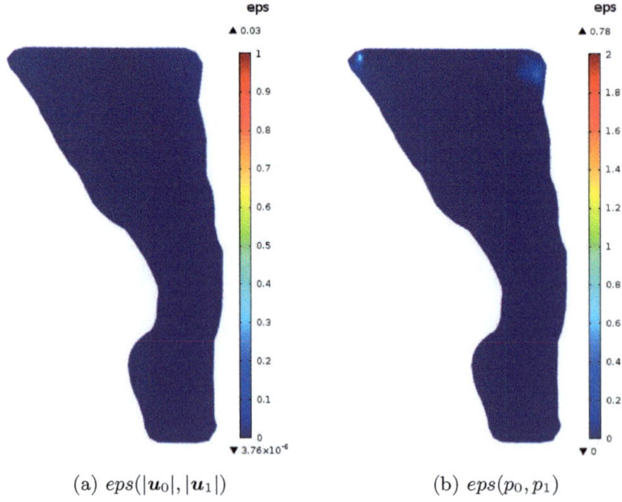

(a) $eps(|\boldsymbol{u}_0|, |\boldsymbol{u}_1|)$ (b) $eps(p_0, p_1)$

Figure 7.16: Difference for the axial slice for the patient without MAA in the simulation with the $k - \epsilon$ turbulence model and boundary condition type two and 20 % decreased reference velocity scale at the inlet.

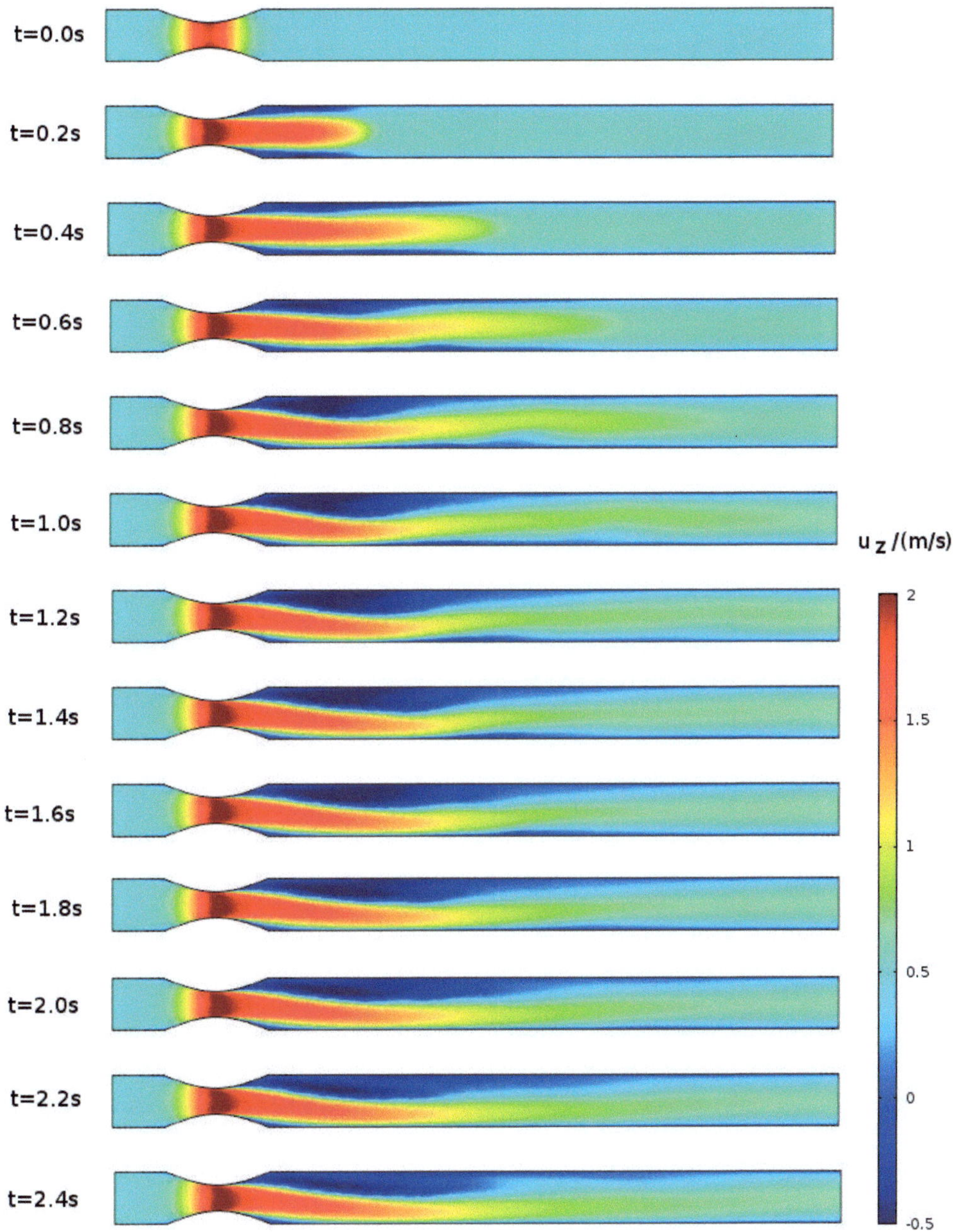

Figure 7.17: Flow simulation for the mesh with 260,675 elements from time $t = 0\,\mathrm{s}$ to $t = 2.4\,\mathrm{s}$.

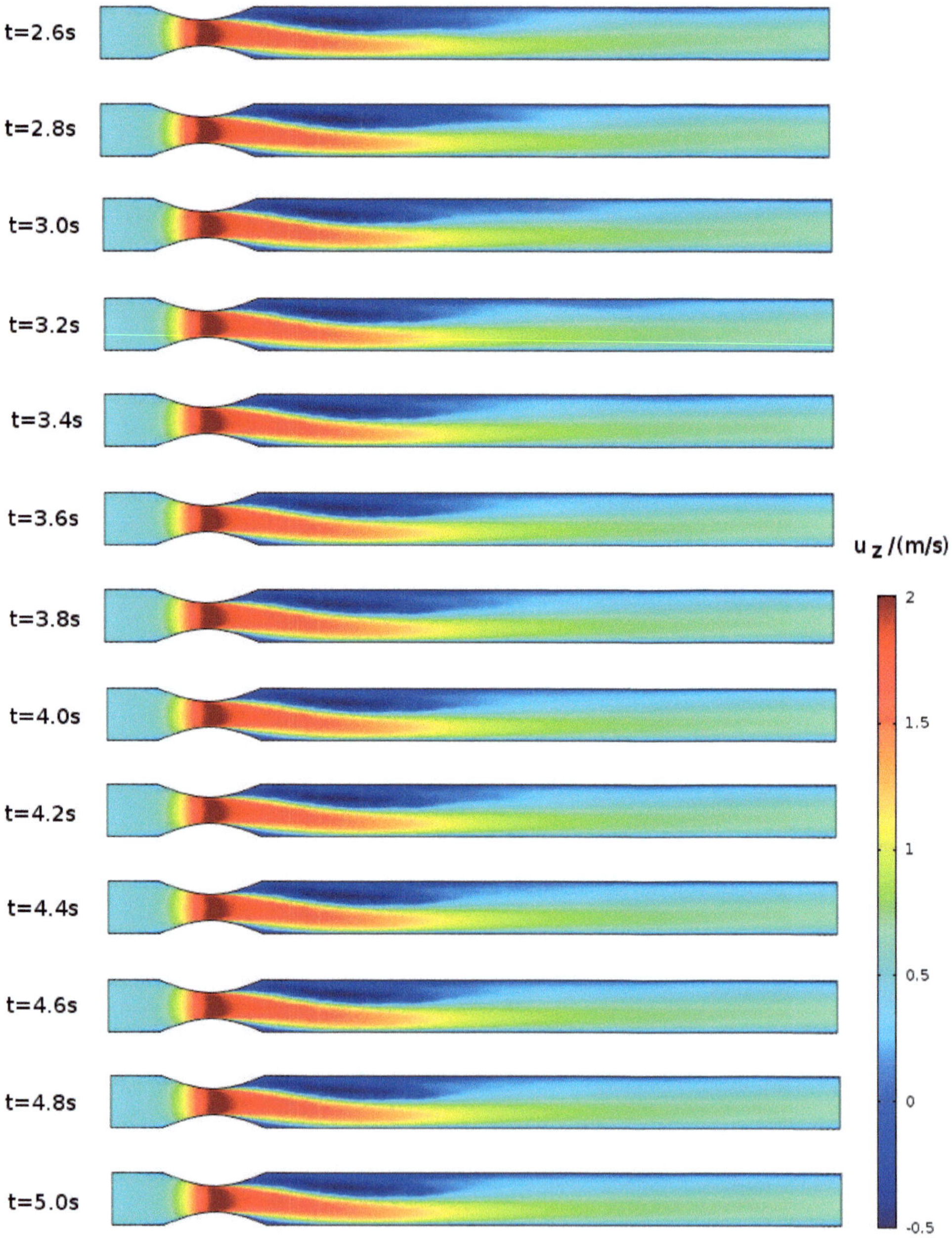

Figure 7.18: Flow simulation for the mesh with 260,675 elements from time $t = 2.6\,\text{s}$ to $t = 5\,\text{s}$.

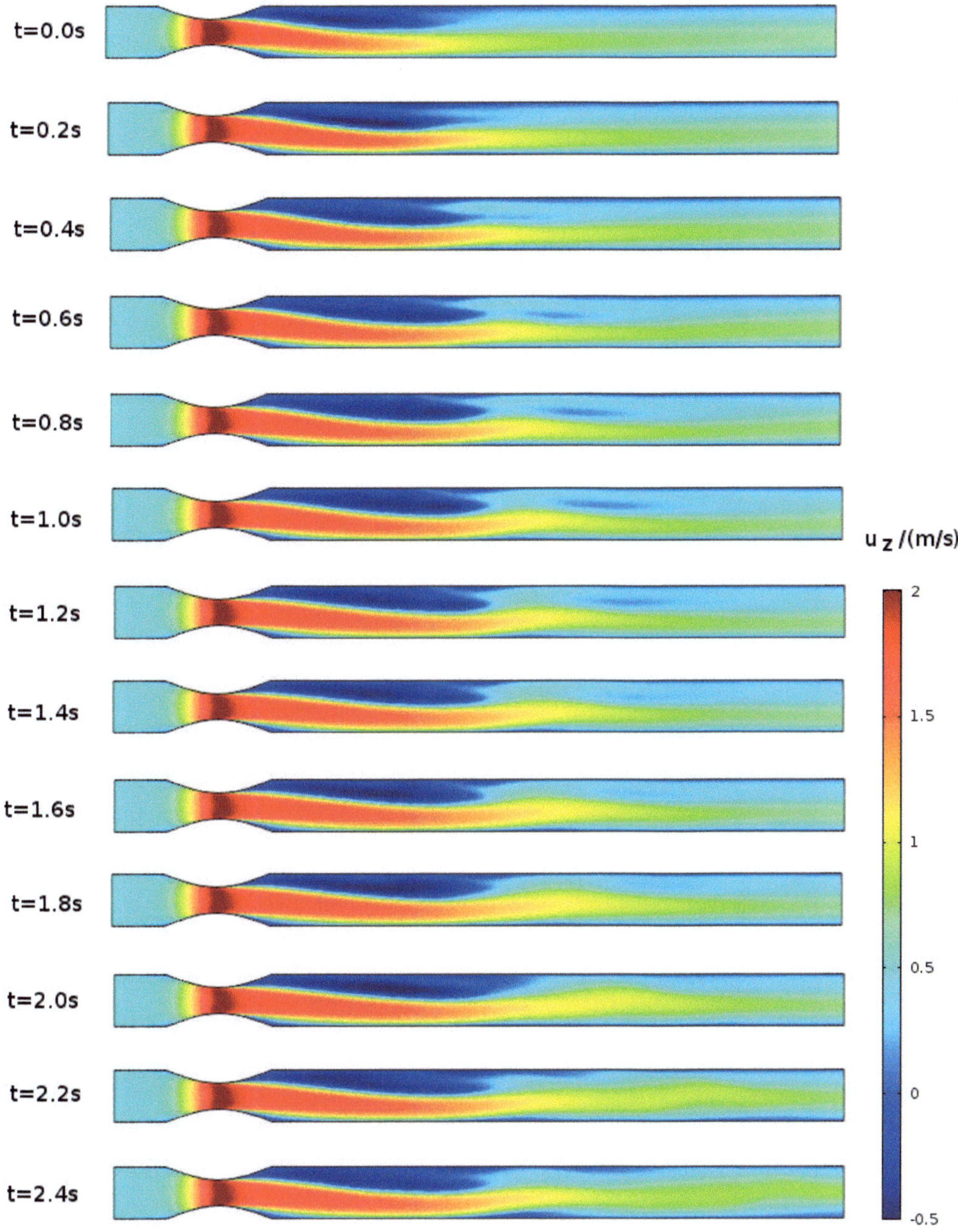

Figure 7.19: Flow simulation for the mesh with 697,212 elements from time $t = 0\,\mathrm{s}$ to $t = 2.4\,\mathrm{s}$.

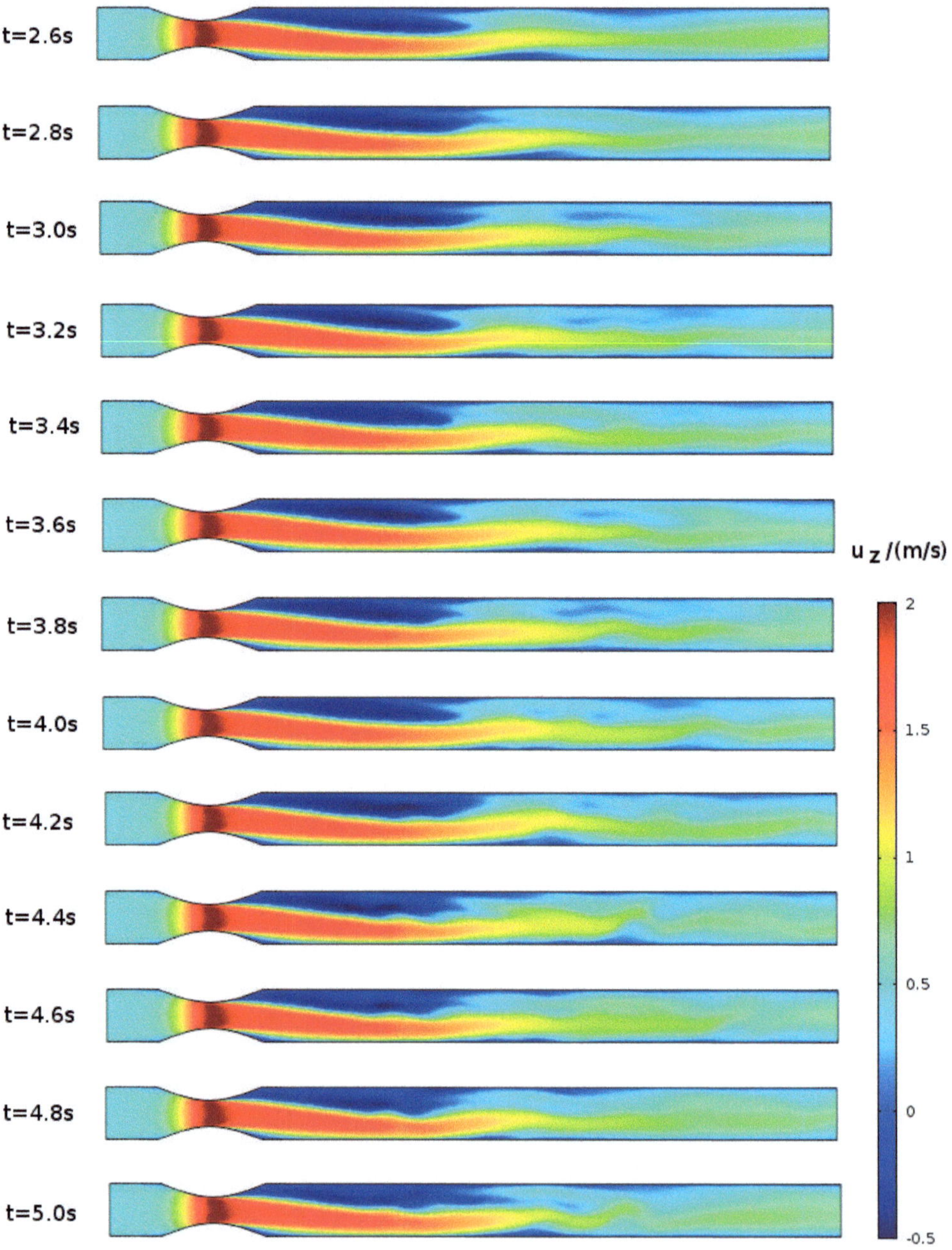

Figure 7.20: Flow simulation for the mesh with 697,212 elements from time $t = 2.6\,$s to $t = 5\,$s.

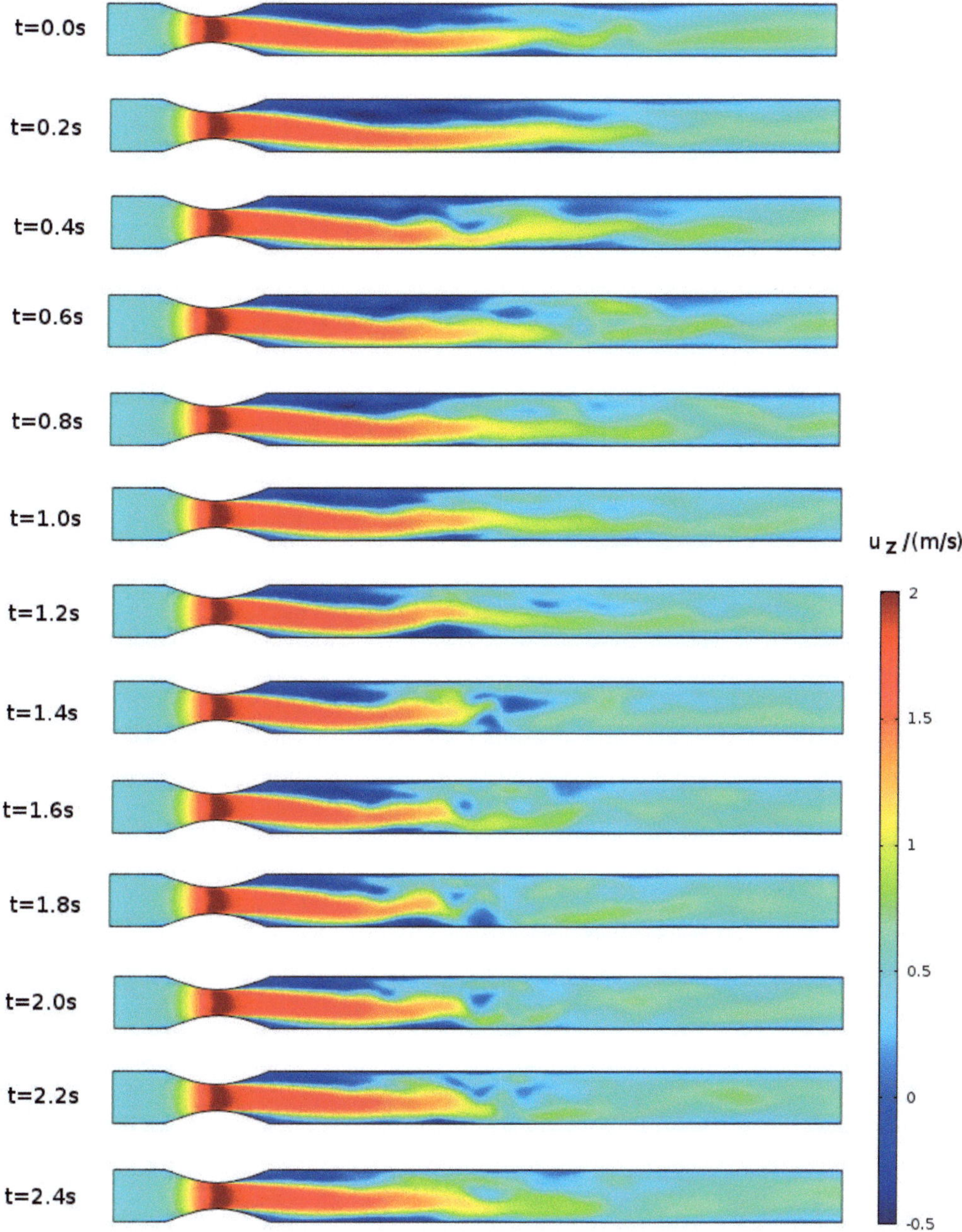

Figure 7.21: Flow simulation for the mesh with 857,360 elements from time $t = 0\,\mathrm{s}$ to $t = 2.4\,\mathrm{s}$.

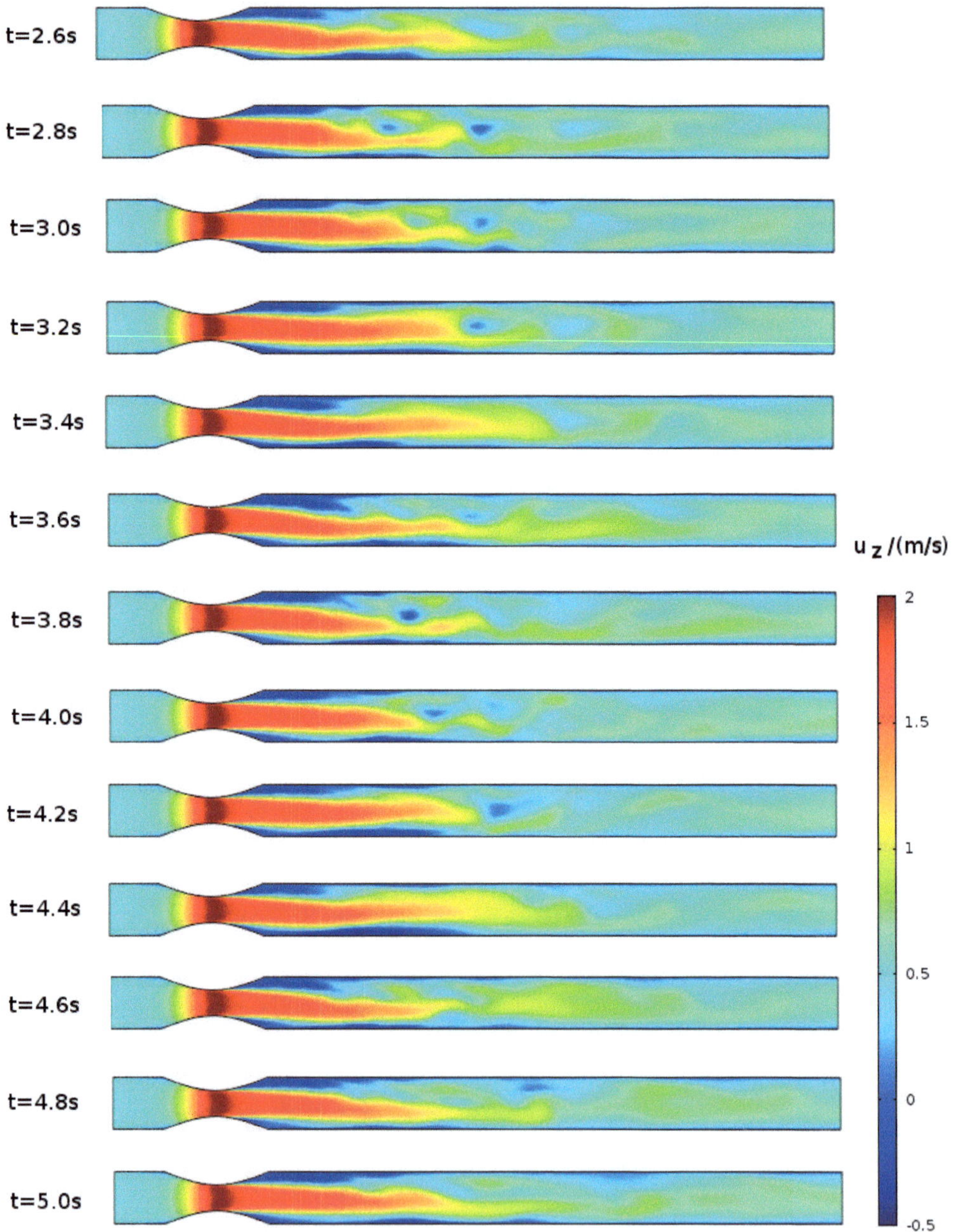

Figure 7.22: Flow simulation for the mesh with 857,360 elements from time $t = 2.6\,\mathrm{s}$ to $t = 5\,\mathrm{s}$.

References

[1] K Abe, T Kondoh, and Y Nagano. A new turbulence model for predicting fluid flow and heat transfer in seperating and reattaching flows. - i. flow field calculations. *International Journal of Heat and Mass Transfer*, 37(1):139–151, 1994.

[2] SA Ahmed and DP Giddens. Velocity measurements in steady flow through axisymmetric stenoses at moderate reynolds numbers. *Journal of Biomechanics*, 16(7):505–516, 1983.

[3] American Academy of Sleep Medicine. *International classification of sleep disorders, revised: Diagnostic and coding manual*. American Academy of Sleep Medicine, Chicago, Illinois, 2001.

[4] American Academy of Sleep Medicine Task Force. Sleep-related breathing disorders in adults: recommendations for syndrome definition and measurement techniques in clinical research. *Sleep*, 22(5):667–689, 1999.

[5] WE Arnoldi. The principle of minimized iteration in the solution of the matrix eigenvalue problem. *Quarterly of Applied Math*, 9:17–29, 1951.

[6] M Benzi. Preconditioning techniques for large linear systems: a survey. *Journal of Computational Physics*, 182:418–477, 2002.

[7] G Bettega, JL Pepin, D Veale, C Deschaux, B Raphaël, and P Lévy. Obstructive sleep apnea syndrome. *American Journal of Respiratory and Critical Care Medicine*, 162:641–649, 2000.

[8] A Boudewyns, M Marklund, and W Hochban. Alternatives for osahs treatment: selection of patients for upper airway surgery and oral appliances. *European Respiratory Review*, 16(106):132–145, 2007.

[9] SC Brenner and C Carstensen. *Finite Element Methods*, volume 1 of *Fundamentals*. John Wiley & Sons, Hoboken, 2004.

[10] W Briggs, VE Henson, and SF McCormick. *A multigrid tutorial*. Society of Industrial and Applied Mathematics, Philadelphia, 2000.

[11] WL Briggs, VE Henson, and SF McCormick. *A multigrid tutorial*. Society for Industrial and Applied Mathematics, Philadelphia, second edition, 2000.

[12] AN Brooks and TJR Hughes. Streamline upwind/petrov-galerkin formulations for convection dominated flows with particular emphasis on the incompressible navier-stokes equations. *Computer Methods in Applied Mechanics and Engineering*, 32:199–259, 1982.

[13] PN Brown, HC Hindmarsh, and LR Petzold. Using krylov methods in the solution of large-scale differential-algebraic systems. *SIAM Journal on Scientific Computing*, 15:1467–1488, 1994.

References

[14] W Cheney and D Kincaid. *Numerical Mathematics and Computing*. Thomson Higher Education, Belmont, sixth edition, 2008.

[15] PY Chou. On the velocity correlations and the solution of the equations of turbulent fluctuation. *Quarterly of Applied Mathematics*, 3:38, 1945.

[16] P Ciarlet. *Lectures on the finite element method*. Tata Institute of Fundamental Research, Bombay, 1975.

[17] WE Lorensen HE Cline. Marching cubes: A high resolution 3d surface construction algorithm. *Computer Graphics*, 21:163–169, 1987.

[18] COMSOL Inc. *COMSOL Multiphysics Reference Guide*, 2013. version 4.4.

[19] D de Zélicourt, K Pekkan, H Kitajima, D Frakes, and AP Yoganathan. Single-step stereolithography of complex anatomical models for optical flow measurements. *Journal of Biomechanical Engineering*, 127(1):204–207, 2005.

[20] BI Davidov. On the statistical dynamics of an incompressible fluid. *Doklady Akademiya Nauk SSSR*, 136:47, 1961.

[21] MA DeLong and JM Ortega. Sor as a preconditioner. *Applied Numerical Mathematics*, 18:431–440, 1995.

[22] P Deuflhard. A modified newton method for the solution of ill-conditioned systems of nonlinear equations with apllication to multiple shooting. *Numerische Mathematik*, 22:289–315, 1974.

[23] DM Driver and HL Seegmiller. Features of a reattaching turbulent shear layer in diverging channel flow. *AIAA Journal*, 23(2):162–171, 1985.

[24] DJ Eckert and A Malhotra. Pathophysiology of adult obstructice sleep apnea. *Proceedings of the American Thoracic Society*, 5(2):144–153, 2008.

[25] LC Evans. *Partial differential equations*, volume 19. American Mathematical Society, Providence, 1998.

[26] Y Fan, LK Cheung, MM Chong, HD Chua, KW Chow, and CH Liu. Computational fluid dynamics analysis on the upper airways of obstructive sleep apnea using patient specific models. *IAENG International Journal of Computer Science*, 38(4), 2013.

[27] JH Ferziger and M Perić. *Computational methods for fluid dynamics*. Springer, Berlin, third edition, 2002.

[28] WH Finlay, KW Stapleton, and J Yokota. On the use of computational fluid dynamics for simulating flow and particle decomposition in the human respiratory tract. *Journal of Aerosol Medicine*, 9(3):329–341, 1996.

[29] M Garland and PS Heckbert. Surface simplification using quadric error metrics. *SIGGRAPH '97: Proceedings of the 24th annual conference on Computer graphics and interactive techniques*, pages 209–216, 1997.

[30] Glycerine Producers' Association. *Physical Properties of Glycerine and Its Solutions*. Glycerine Producers' Association, 1963.

[31] W Hackbusch. *Theorie und Numerik elliptischer Differentialgleichungen.* Teubner Studienbücher, Stuttgart, 1986.

[32] J Hadamard. Sur les problmes aux drives partielles et leur signification physique. *Princeton University Bulletin*, pages 49–52, 1902.

[33] FH Harlow and PI Nakayama. Transport of turbulence energy decay rate. *Los Alamos Science Laboratory, University of California*, 1968. Report LA-3854.

[34] AF Heenan, E Matida, A Pollard, and WH Finlay. Experimental measurements and computational modeling of the flow field in an idealized human oropharynx. *Experiments in Fluids*, 35:70–84, 2003.

[35] AC Hindmarsh, PN Brown, KE Grant, SL Lee, R Serban, DE Shumaker, and CS Woodward. Sundials: Suite of nonlinear and differential/algebraic equation solvers. *ACM Transactions on Mathematical Software*, 21(2):363–396, 2005.

[36] COMSOL Inc. www.comsol.com.

[37] V John and P Knobloch. On spurious oscillations at layers diminishing (sold) methods for convection – diffusion equations: Part i – a review. *Computer Methods in Applied Mechanics and Engineering*, 196:2197–2215, 2007.

[38] V John and G Matthies. Higher-order finite element discretization in a benchmark problem for incompressible flows. *International Journal for Numerical Methods in Fluids*, 40:775–798, 2001.

[39] JW De Backer, OM Vanderveken, WG Vos, A Devolder, SL Verhulst, JA Verbraecken, PM Parizel, MJ Braem, PH Van de Heyning, and WA de Backer. Functional imaging using computational fluid dynamics to predict treatment success of mandibular advancement devices in sleep-disordered breathing. *Journal of Biomechanics*, 40(16):3708–3714, 2007.

[40] T Keck, R Leiacker, H Riechelmann, and G Rettinger. Temperature profile in the nasal cavity. *The Laryngoscope*, 110:615–654, 2000.

[41] R R Kerswell. Recent progress in understanding the transition to turbulence in a pipe. *Nonlinearity*, 18:R17–R44, 2005.

[42] AN Kolmogorov. Local structure of turbulence in incompressible viscous fluid for very large reynolds number. *Doklady Akademiya Nauk SSSR*, 30:299–303, 1941.

[43] AN Kolmogorov. Equations of turbulent motion of an incompressible fluid. *Izvestia Academy of Science, USSR; Physics*, 6:56–58, 1942.

[44] D Kuzmin and O Mierka. On the implementation of the $k - \epsilon$ turbulence model in incompressible flow solvers based on a finite element discretization. *International Journal of Computing Science and Mathematics*, 1(2–4):193–206, 2007.

[45] BE Launder and BI Sharma. Application of energy dissipation model of turbulence to the calculation of flow near a spinning disc. *Letters in Heat and Mass Transfer*, 1(2):131–138, 2013.

[46] P Lavie, P Herer, and V Hoffstein. Obstructive sleep apnoea syndrome as a risk factor for hypertension: population study. *BMJ*, 320:479–482, 2000.

References

[47] LC Lawrence. *Partial Differential Equations*. American Mathematical Society, Providence, 1998.

[48] HF Li, ZF Tian, JY Tu, W Yang, GH Yeoh, CL Xue, and CG Li. Studies of airflow through a human nasopharynx and pharynx airway. *Proceedings of the 5th International Conference on CFD in the Process Industries*, 2006.

[49] JY Lu, JH Hong, CY Wang, KZ Lee, and HC Yang. Measurements and simulation of turbulent flow in a steep open-channel with smooth boundary. *Journal of the Chinese Institute of Engineers*, 26(2):201–210, 2003.

[50] TB Martonen, Z Zhang, and RC Lessmann. Fluid dynamics of the human larynx and upper tracheobronchial airways. *Aerosol Science and Technology*, 19(2):133–156, 1993.

[51] MeVis Medical Solutions AG and Fraunhofer MEVIS. *MeVisLab*. Bremen. software available: http://www.mevislab.de/.

[52] F Meyer. Topographic distance and watershed lines. *Signal Processing*, 38:113–125, 1994.

[53] M Mihaescu, S Murugappan, E Gutmark, LF Donnelly, S Khosla, and M Kalra. Computational fluid dynamics analysis of upper airway reconstructed from magnetic resonance imaging data. *Annals of Otology, Rhinology and Laryngology*, 117(4):303–309, 2008.

[54] RS Monteroa, IM Llorente, and MD Salas. Robust multigrid algorithms for the navier–stokes equations. *Journal of Computational Physics*, 173(2):412–432, 2001.

[55] H Oertel jr., editor. *Prandtl - Führer durch die Strömungslehre*. Vieweg, Braunschweig, eleventh edition, 2002.

[56] OpenStax College. Organs and structures of the respiratory system. *Connexions*, Jul 8, 2013. Accessed: 02.08.13.

[57] PE Peppard, T Young, M Palta, and J Skatrud. Prospective study of the association between sleep-disordered breathing and hypertension. *The New England Journal of Medicine*, 342(19):1378–1384, 2000.

[58] MA Puhan, A Suarez, CL Cascio, A Zahn, M Heitz, and O Braendli. Didgeridoo playing as alternative treatment for obstructive sleep apnoea syndrome: randomised controlled trial. *British Medical Journal*, 332:266–270, 2006.

[59] A Quarteroni, R Sacco, and F Saleri. *Numerical mathematics*. Springer Verlag, Berlin, second edition, 2007.

[60] JF Ramirez, E Mesa, JW Branch, and P Boulanger. A comparison between lagrange multiplier and penalty methods for setting boundary conditions in mesh-free methods. *Revista Avances en Sistemas e Informática*, 8(3):51–56, 2011.

[61] MR Rasani, K Inthavong, and JY Tu. Simulation of pharyngeal airway interaction with air flow using low-re turbulencemodel. *Modelling and Simulation in Engineering*, 2011, 2011.

[62] M Renardy and RC Rogers. *An introduction to partial differential equations*. Number 13 in Texts in Applied Mathematics. Springer-Verlag, New York, second edition, 2004.

[63] CM Ryan and TD Bradley. Pathogenesis of obstructive sleep apnea. *Journal of Applied Physiology*, 99:2440–2450, 2005.

[64] J Saad and MH Schultz. Gmres: A generalized minimal residual algorithm for solving non-symmetric linear systems. *SIAM Journal of Scientific and Statistical Computing*, 7(3):856–869, 1986.

[65] O Schenk. Pardiso project. *http://www.pardiso-project.org/*, 2013. accessed: 07.12.13.

[66] O Schenk, K Gärtner, W Fichtner, and A Stricker. Pardiso: a high-performance serial and parallel sparse linear solver in semiconductor device simulation. *Future Generation Computer Systems*, 18(1):69–78, 2001.

[67] CM Schroeder and R O'Hara. Depression and obstructive sleep apnea (osa). *Annals of General Psychiatry*, 4(13), 2005.

[68] HR Schwarz. *Methode der finiten Elemente*. Teubner Studienbücher, Stuttgart, third edition, 1991.

[69] B Shome, LP Wang, MH Santare, AK Prasad, AZ Szeri, and D Roberts. Modeling of airflow in the pharynx with application to sleep apnea. *Journal of Biomedical Engineering*, 120:416–422, 1998.

[70] Sicat GmbH & Co. KG. http://www.sicat.com/en.html.

[71] H Sigloch. *Technische Fluidmechanik*. Springer, Berlin, sixth edition, 2008.

[72] GI Taylor. Statistical theory of turbulence. *Proceedings of the Royal Society*, A151:421, 1935.

[73] C van Holsbeke, J de Baker, W Vos, P Verdonck, P van Ransbeeck, T Claessens, M Braem O Vanderveken, and W de Baker. Anatomical and functional changes in the upper airways of sleep apnea patients due to mandibular repositioning: A large scale study. *Journal of Biomechanics*, 44:442–449, 2011.

[74] W Vos, J De Backer, A Devolder, O Vanderveken, S Verhulst, R Salgado, P Germonpre, B Partoens, F Wuyts, P Parizel, and W De Backer. Correlation between severity of sleep apnea and upper airway morphology based on advanced anatomical and functional imaging. *Journal of Biomechanics*, 40:2207–2213, 2007.

[75] COMSOL© W. Frei. *Which turbulence model should I use for my CFD application*. 2013. http://www.comsol.com/blogs/which-turbulence-model-should-choose-cfd-application/, accessed: 23.11.13.

[76] DC Wilcox. *Turbulence modeling for CFD*. DCW Industries, La Cañada, second edition, 1998.

[77] C Xu, S Sin, JM McDonough, JK Udupa A Guez, R Arens, and DM Wootton. Computational fluid dynamics modeling of the upper airway of children with obstructive sleep apena syndrome in steady flow. *Journal of Biomechanics*, 39(11):2043–2054, 2006.

[78] D Xun. On the weak discontinuity surfaces and tapes of equation systems in fluid mechanics. *Acta Mathematicae Applicatae Sinica*, 4(1):75–82, 1988.

[79] HK Yaggi, J Concato, W Kernan, JH Lichtman, LM Brass, and V Mohsenin. Obstructive sleep apnea as a risk factor for stroke and death. *The New England Journal of Medicine*, 353:2034–2041, 2005.

References

[80] T Young, M Palta, J Dempsey, J Skatrud, S Weber, and S Badr. The occurrence of sleep-disordered breathing among middle-aged adults. *The New England Journal Of Medicine*, 328(17):1230–1235, 1993.

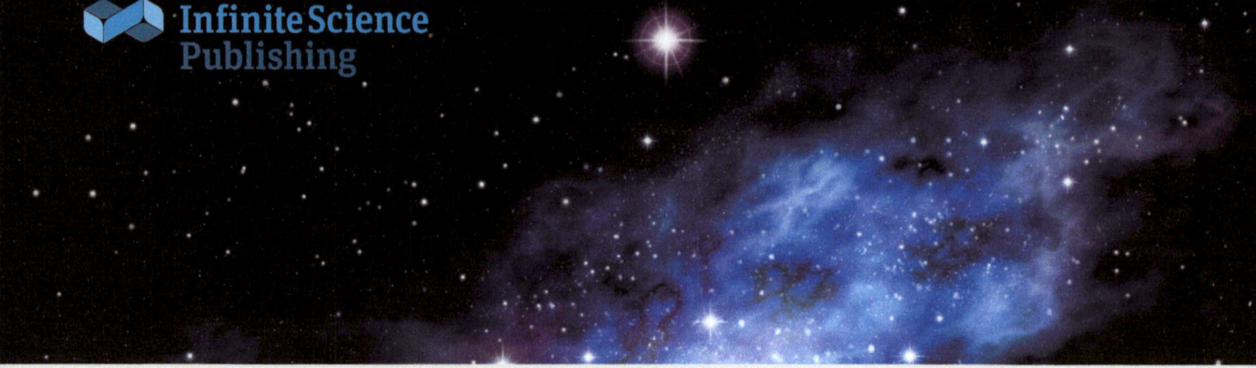